true FOOD

8 Simple Steps to a Healthier You

ANNIE B. BOND • MELISSA BREYER • WENDY GORDON

NATIONAL GEOGRAPHIC
WASHINGTON, D.C.

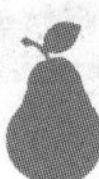

To all the people whose hands reach out to sow the seed,
till the soil, pick the produce, snap the beans,
remove the stems, and make the meal.

Contents

Foreword

By Alice Waters, ***owner and founder of Chez Panisse***

Growing, cooking, and sharing food with friends has always been the most important aspect of my life. My first taste memories were family dinners of fresh corn, green beans, and strawberries picked right out of my parents' victory garden. For me, the daily ritual of the table gives life meaning and beauty. Mealtime is the place where we pass the peas and learn about generosity. It is the place where you share a plate and where you truly learn about somebody else: You practice empathy.

Unfortunately, studies show that over 85 percent of Americans no longer eat even one meal at home together every day. When Annie B. Bond, Melissa Breyer, and Wendy Gordon write about going "out of true" in this invaluable book, I am reminded of how seriously our nation has veered out of alignment, especially in the ways we grow, buy, eat, and think about food.

Eating "true" is something that's natural to everyone on this planet, yet with fast food omnipresent in our lives, we've abandoned our traditions and basic knowledge. How, then, can we come back to the table and back to our senses? Well, I've always been an idealist—some might say downright uncompromising when it comes to the way I think food should be produced and consumed. That's why it's my pleasure to introduce this practical guide, *True Food.* In it, we're fed thoughtful how-tos on everything from stocking a pantry to preserving the harvest through the seasons to composting what you can't use. Most important, *True Food* demonstrates the value of buying locally and organically grown food.

I learned these lessons in 1971, when I started Chez Panisse in Berkeley, California. At first I was only looking for flavor, not philosophy. I wanted tiny, juicy raspberries; succulent sweet peppers; and lamb that tasted of grass and sunlight. In my quest to find local Northern Californian ingredients reminiscent of the vibrant flavors of France, I discovered that farmers and ranchers who cared for the land and practiced organic techniques produced the most beautiful and delicious food. Now 85 suppliers provide Chez Panisse with ingredients throughout the year.

When I began shopping at farmers' markets and getting to know the people behind the food, I began to think of myself as a co-producer. By choosing to buy food grown locally and sustainably, I was weaving myself into a community that shares an appreciation for the value of food itself and how it connects us to time and place, the seasons, and the natural cycle. As the Slow Food Manifesto explains, we must remain "in true" within the subtle balance of our right to pleasure and our responsibility to our heritage of food, tradition, and culture. With this book in hand, you can begin to cultivate the connection between plate and planet. *True Food: 8 Simple Steps to a Healthier You* will help you and your family nourish yourselves—deliciously!

Introduction

How we eat determines to a considerable extent how the world is used. **—WENDELL BERRY, FARMER AND POET**

A simple September supper including local, sweet, vine-ripened tomatoes, freshly picked corn, and miraculously ripe peaches grown nearby with organic local cream on top is a meal one savors forever. Much of the reason is that such a meal is made up of real food with true flavor, food that isn't produced with a priority of yield, market appeal, shelf life, and durability, but food grown in living soil with health and stewardship in mind, from farms that include heritage livestock breeds and heirloom varieties of produce for preserving genetic diversity.

Home-cooked meals using locally harvested food are uplifting to us on every level: They are nourishing, flavorful, and sensual—and they connect us to the ground and community where we live. Eating a diet of such food works on behalf of the environment as well as on behalf of our bodies, senses, and spirit. It integrates the innovative flavors of greenmarket cuisine with its wide range of healthful nutrients and antioxidants, the pure joy of eating, and the unique and pressing concerns about stewardship and sustainability of Earth's resources.

How many of us know this sort of food, or this way of eating? Half of the population? A quarter? Less? You may have heard the phrase "out of true." It means not in correct alignment. During the last 40 years or so, most of us have been eating a diet that is wildly out of true compared to what our bodies need, and equally out of true considering what is best for the health of the planet.

When we consider our Earth system, which is itself so out of true, we might first think of climate, which scientists overwhelmingly agree has been knocked off track by global warming. But global warming is the consequence of other systems that are themselves out of true, our energy production system being the most significant. We get far too much of our energy from the burning of fossil fuels, which puts CO_2 and other greenhouse gases into the atmosphere, leading to climate change and a planet out of true. No surprise, but our fossil fuel–dependent food system is out of true as well, not aligned to either our health or our environment.

People themselves are energy burners. Food is our fuel, and the harm of a food supply system spinning off course is evident in the high percentage of Americans who are overweight and diabetic, the water supplies that are contaminated, the rain forests that are destroyed, and the global warming gases produced as we work to sustain our global food network.

There are many people and groups today working to get the food system back in true alignment, working to preserve and sustain "true food," but we—the food shoppers and eaters—are the most important.

"Me?" you say. "Can I really make a difference to improve what we eat and protect the planet?" Yes! That's why we wrote *True Food,* to be a primer, a tool kit, a simple set of steps that will take you and how you eat in a new direction, and bring you, your health, and the planet all back into line. It's simpler, cheaper, and more pleasing than you think, since *True Food* is really all about getting back to basics, about restoring what's good about food, reconnecting with real food, whole food, food that's local, and supporting and sustaining those food systems that put health first, starting with the soil and not stopping until the plate.

True Food will help you find, or find again, the pleasures you may still remember about food, the flavors packed in a fresh tomato, the delights of home-grown, the healthfulness abundant in home-cooked. The amazing thing is, by embracing the steps set forth in *True Food,* you will find that things really do start falling into place. On the most basic cellular level, your body will begin to feel more in tune, echoing in microcosm the effects that your food choices have on your family, your home, your community, and the planet. The simple choice to select, cook, serve, and eat true food can help ease these realms back into alignment, bringing it all back in to true.

STEP 1

Eat Local Food

Eat locally: Do it to decrease energy consumption; do it to support producers in your region, many of whom are leaders in the conservation of open space, water quality, wildlife, and local food traditions; do it for the flavor! Step away from big-business produce (grown far away and selected for ease of transport and a long shelf life) and opt for the healthy, true flavors of locally grown food. Do it for the sense of place and to strengthen ties within your community.

WHAT IT MEANS

Eating Locally

Be mindful of how far food travels to get to you.

The most commonsense way of stating this principle is: The shorter the distance that food travels from farm to table, the better. Simply consider the distance between you and your food sources (and we're not talking supermarkets here—they're vendors, not sources), and choose the closest producers. Get your eggs from a farm in your town rather than from a farm in the far reaches of your state, and vegetables from farms in your state rather than from farms two states over. If you live on the East Coast, Florida citrus is better than California citrus. If you live in the state of Washington, California is closer than Florida, but Florida is closer than Brazil, and so forth.

***The Oxford American Dictionary* named "locavore" as the 2007 Word of the Year.**

Eating locally doesn't mean doing without. You don't have to give up coffee and tea, for example, which are popular the world over, though grown only in certain regions. But it does mean making choices when possible in favor of those foods produced nearest to where you live. Every time you purchase from the closest farmer, you strengthen the network of growers and businesses seeking to build and maintain a "foodshed" that is diverse, nutritious, sustainable, and secure.

The need to maintain the local foodshed has been a matter of concern for almost a century. In 1929, urban planner Walter Hedden in *How Great Cities Are Fed* first introduced the idea of a foodshed—the geographic area embracing consumers and the producers of the food they consume. Hedden was prompted to write about foodsheds when nationwide railroad transportation was threatened in October 1921. Fifty-some years later, the concept of "eating locally" was reintroduced, again in response to transportation concerns, and in particular to the oil shocks of the 1970s.

Now, just a decade into the 21st century, climate change and rising energy prices have once again brought our attention to the systems underpinning our national, even international, foodsheds. Many are asking whether local food systems might not provide a more energy-efficient, secure, and sustainable source of food.

Many have picked up on the terms "foodshed" and "eating locally" to advance a vision of how agriculture can thrive in low-density suburban and ex-urban areas by targeting consumers in metropolitan areas. San Francisco–based chef and writer Jessica Prentice coined the term "locavore" to describe and promote the practice of eating food harvested within a 100-mile radius of one's home. Writers Aaron Newton and Sharon Astyk took it a step further and created the idea of the Bull's-eye Diet—a dartboard concept, where your home and what you can grow there is at the center, with each concentric circle representing the increasing distance of your food away from your own home and garden.

Local sourcing doesn't mean one can't maintain an ethnic diet. Vendors in New York City's Chinatown get many of their traditional Chinese vegetables from New Jersey farmers. People who move north from the tropics can easily grow or buy locally grown hot peppers. Culturally appropriate seasonings help a lot to make food taste more familiar.

The long-distance, large-scale transportation of food consumes sizable quantities of fossil fuels. In 1940, it took an average of 1 calorie of fossil-fuel energy to produce 2.3 calories of food energy. Now it takes closer to 7–10 calories of fossil fuel energy to produce every 1 calorie of food energy.

We need a system of decentralized, small-scale industries to transform the products of our fields and woodlands and streams: small creameries, cheese factories, canneries, grain mills, saw mills, furniture factories, and the like.

—WENDELL BERRY, FARMER AND POET

WHY IT MATTERS FOR YOU

Local Flavors, Higher Food Value

Food grown locally is often more nutritious. Tastes better, too.

A wide range of benefits have been attributed to local food. While most of the expected benefits of eating local food are ecological and economical, many also believe that local foods taste better and are more nutritious than foods bred and picked for their ability to endure long-distance shipping.

Experts are now wondering whether a more local food system would decrease food safety risks by decentralizing food production. Joan Gussow, influential nutritionist and author, urges growers to be inventive by extending the seasons and pushing the limits of what they can grow. She herself grows some citrus in her home, just north of New York City. She has lime and lemon trees, and even a grapefruit and an orange tree. Pawpaws, a fruit that tastes like bananas, can live in the North, and she is trying to grow them, too. She welcomes investigations to determine if local greenhouses use less energy than that required to import food from elsewhere, or if solar greenhouses can become a realistic way to grow large amounts of food and extend growing seasons. She notes that "local freezing and food processing are what we really need; we could create a market for frozen local organic food."

The distance from which our food comes represents our separation from the knowledge of how and by whom what we consume is produced, processed, and transported.... Can we stay within a hundred-mile radius? —LOCAVORES.COM

WHAT IT MEANS FOR EARTH

Making a Global Impact

Choosing food that travels a short distance tangibly benefits the environment.

The long-distance transport of food requires more preservatives, packaging, refrigeration, and fuel, and generates huge amounts of waste and pollution every step of the way. Only recently, though, with rising fuel prices and a deepening understanding of the link between fossil-fuel burning and climate change, has the true cost of our far-flung food web become a subject of greater debate. The question experts are now asking is: Would shifts to diets based on more local foods reduce energy use and climate-altering emissions as well as enhance food security?

One thing is certain: Both communities and the environment benefit from a strengthened local food

Fun, Kids, Pleasure

SAVOR YOUR FAVORITES FROM AFAR

Eating locally need not mean you can never eat pineapple, even if you live in Maine.

"For most people," writes Martin Teitel in his book *Rain Forest in Your Kitchen,* "the end of December is a special time: decorations adorn stores, streets, and houses; aromas of fir trees, wood fires, and spiced cider waft through the air; special music, books, and clothes are brought out of closets. Would the holiday be as wonderful if we kept the Christmas tree up all year, opened presents every morning, or had turkey and stuffing for dinner each night?"

In just the same spirit, save pineapple as a treat for a special occasion—especially in the fall, when they are abundant, because that is their season.

system where the supply chain is short and relationships are forged directly between producers and consumers. Under the current global food system, instead of dealing directly with their neighbors, farmers sell into a remote and complex food chain of which they are a tiny part—and they are paid accordingly: Worldwide, farmers typically receive just a few cents of the food dollar. Most of it goes to middlemen (processors, packagers, distributors, and marketers). A whole constellation of relationships within the foodshed—between neighbors, between farmers and local processors, between farmers and consumers—is lost in the process. The supposed efficiencies of the long-distance food web leave many people less well nourished and underserved at both ends of the chain.

Your state department of agriculture can provide information on what's local in your region and where best to shop for local fruit and vegetables.

HOW TO DO IT

Food from Your Neighborhood

Eating locally is easier than you might think—there are many ways to implement a local diet.

One way to start eating local food is by getting to know your nearby farmers' seasons, including how to buy locally in the winter. Cooking with flexibility, depending on what is available, helps a lot, as does learning the difference between local and organic and searching out local farmers and suppliers of organic food. Getting children to eat a local diet can be fun, as can learning how to shop in new ways, such as through community-supported agriculture (CSAs), subscription farming, pick-your-own farms, farmers' market shopping, growing your own food, and collecting wild edibles.

Getting to Know Your Local Seasons

Following a diet of the seasonal harvest is a joy. In the Northeast, spring begins with sweet strawberries and tart rhubarb, a perfect combination; then berries and melons in the summer; and apples, pears, and even peaches in the fall and winter. Apples can be placed in cold storage, still crisp, for use through early spring, when the strawberries come in. Vegetables follow a different pattern, starting with peas and spinach in the spring and moving to parsnips and sweet potatoes for winter stews.

Every region of the country has its harvest seasons, including California and Florida where crops can be grown year-round. The following chart is a start on getting to know what's local and seasonal in your area and meshing your diet with what's in season nearest you. You'll enjoy fruit and vegetables at their peak of ripeness and nutritional value.

And if they don't taste better, we'll eat this book!

Cooking & Eating

PLANT A COOK'S GARDEN

One concept that comes from Aaron Newton and Sharon Astyk's Bull's-eye Diet is to make your garden into a cook's garden. It can be as simple as growing potted heirloom tomatoes or rosemary on the patio—or as complex as creating a garden close to the kitchen door that serves a seasonal menu: spinach and snap peas in spring, salad ingredients all summer long. Over time, you can develop a full year's harvest of vegetables.

You must gather your fruit when it is Ripe, and not before, else will it wither, and be tough and sowr.

—WILLIAM LAWSON, *THE COUNTRY HOUSEWIFE'S GARDEN* (1617)

What's in Season? A Guide to Local Eating in the United States

The Northeast

Late Spring

FRUIT Rhubarb, strawberries

VEGETABLES Asparagus, mushrooms (cultivated), peas, spinach

Summer

FRUIT Blackberries, blueberries, boysenberries, cherries, currants, raspberries, strawberries

VEGETABLES Beans (snap), celery, corn, cucumbers, eggplant, endive, escarole, fennel, kale, kohlrabi, lettuce, mushrooms, onions, peppers, radishes, summer squash, tomatoes, watercress

Fall

FRUIT Apples, cantaloupes, grapes, honeydew melons, peaches, pears, plums, quince, watermelons

VEGETABLES Acorn squash, beans, beets, broccoli, Brussels sprouts, cabbage, carrots, cauliflower, celeriac, celery, corn, eggplant, garlic, Jerusalem artichokes, kale, leeks, onions, parsnips, potatoes, pumpkins, rabe, rutabaga, winter squash

Winter

FRUIT From root cellars and cold storage: apples, pears

VEGETABLES From root cellars and cold storage: beets, cabbage, carrots, leeks, onions, parsnips, potatoes, pumpkins, sweet potatoes, turnips, winter squash

The South

Spring

FRUIT Strawberries, blueberries, peaches, watermelon, melons, cantaloupes, boysenberries, cherries

VEGETABLES Carrots, greens, snap peas, onions, yellow squash, zucchini, cabbage, sweet corn, tomatoes, bell peppers, cucumbers, scallions, summer squash, asparagus, broccoli

Summer

FRUIT Blueberries, cantaloupes, watermelons, apples, peaches, grapes, muscadines, apricots, figs, boysenberries, nectarines, gooseberries, Asian pears, raspberries

VEGETABLES Carrots, greens, snap peas, onions, yellow squash, zucchini, cabbage, sweet corn, tomatoes, cucumbers, field peas, butter beans, peppers, scallions, potatoes, eggplant, beets, beans

Fall

FRUIT Apples, watermelons

VEGETABLES Cucumbers, field peas, greens, snap beans, sweet corn, sweet potatoes, yellow squash, zucchini, bell peppers, cabbage, tomatoes, pumpkins, winter squash, Brussels sprouts

Winter

FRUIT Apples, oranges, grapefruit, lemons, tangerines, tangelos

VEGETABLES Carrots, greens, sweet potatoes

The Midwest

Spring

FRUIT Strawberries, rhubarb

VEGETABLES Spinach, kohlrabi, asparagus, broccoli, cabbage

Summer

FRUIT Berries, watermelon, apples, peaches, figs, pears

VEGETABLES Broccoli, cabbage, carrots, cauliflower, collards, cucumber, daikon, eggplant, garlic, green beans, hot peppers, kale, leeks, lettuce, mushrooms, onions, peas, radishes, rhubarb, salad greens, scallions, shallots, spinach, summer squash, sweet corn, sweet peppers, tomatoes, chard, turnips, string beans, corn, potatoes

Fall

FRUIT Raspberries, apples, cranberries

VEGETABLES Cabbage, gourds, pumpkins, turnips, snow peas, kohlrabi, leeks, brussels sprouts, winter squash

Winter

FRUIT From cold storage: apples

VEGETABLES Cabbage, gourds; from cold storage: potatoes

The Northwest

Spring

FRUIT Boysenberries, cherries, strawberries, rhubarb

VEGETABLES Asparagus, greens, onions, garlic, collard greens, carrots, mushrooms, cauliflower, peas

Summer

FRUIT Berries, cherries, apricots, rhubarb, nectarines

VEGETABLES Asparagus, beans, beets, broccoli, cabbage, carrots, celery, cucumber, eggplant, greens, peas, summer squash, tomatoes, peppers, potatoes, winter squash, sweet corn

Fall

FRUIT Apples, pears, raspberries, nectarines, peaches, blueberries

VEGETABLES Beans, beets, broccoli, Brussels sprouts, cabbage, carrots, cucumbers, eggplant, greens, peppers, potatoes, pumpkins, summer squash, sweet corn, tomatoes, winter squash

Winter

FRUIT From cold storage: apples

VEGETABLES From cold storage: potatoes

The Southwest

Spring

FRUIT Apricots

VEGETABLES Salad greens, asparagus, peas, radishes, spinach

Summer

FRUIT Apples, melons, peaches, pears, berries, figs, cherries, raspberries, plums, blackberries, grapes, watermelons, nectarines

VEGETABLES Summer squash, sweet corn, black-eyed peas, cucumbers, green beans, okra, white tamale corn, bell peppers, tomatoes, potatoes, spinach, beets, chili peppers, garlic, broccoli, carrots, tomatillos, onions, eggplant

Fall

FRUIT Apples, peaches, pears, berries

VEGETABLES Pumpkins, winter squash, potatoes, sweet potatoes, tomatillos, red chili peppers, bell peppers

Winter

FRUIT Apples

VEGETABLES Pumpkins, winter squash, potatoes

California

Spring

FRUIT Avocados, bananas, cherries, grapefruit, lemons, mangoes, navel oranges, papaya, pineapple, plums, rhubarb, strawberries

VEGETABLES Artichokes, asparagus, broccoli, cabbage, cauliflower, celery, cucumbers, garlic, leeks, lettuce, mushrooms, onions, peas, potatoes, rhubarb, snap beans, spinach, squash, watercress

Summer

FRUIT Apricots, blueberries, boysenberries, cantaloupe, grapefruit, grapes, lemons, melons, nectarines, peaches, strawberries, Valencia oranges, watermelons

VEGETABLES Artichokes, cabbage, carrots, cauliflower, celery, corn, cucumbers, eggplant, garlic, bell peppers, kohlrabi, lettuce, mushrooms, okra, onions, potatoes, spinach, squash, tomatoes, watercress

Fall

FRUIT Apples, cantaloupes, cranberries, dates, grapefruit, grapes, melons, lemons, kiwi, papayas, pears, persimmons

VEGETABLES Artichokes, broccoli, cabbage, carrots, cauliflower, celery, chili peppers, corn, cucumbers, dry beans, endive, escarole, bell peppers, leeks, lettuce, onions, parsnips, peas, potatoes, squash, rutabaga, spinach, sweet potatoes, turnips

Winter

FRUIT Grapefruit, lemons, kiwi, navel oranges, persimmons, tangelos, tangerines

VEGETABLES Artichokes, broccoli, Brussels sprouts, carrots, cauliflower, celery, lettuce, mushrooms, potatoes, rutabaga, spinach, squash, tomatoes, turnips

HOW TO BUY LOCAL IN WINTER Out-of-season produce is an extravagance because it is so energy-intensive to transport it to your kitchen. It's not just your drive to bring it home from the grocery store—think of all the traveling that produce has done to get to the store from whatever field or orchard it was grown in. But you still want to eat plenty of fruit and vegetables, so in the winter, we should all try to eat frozen, dried, and bisphenol A (BPA)-free canned food, and food stored in local root cellars.

Eating frozen fruit and vegetables, especially from local producers and local root cellars, is your very best option during the winter months. Frozen foods retain much of their nutritional content, in addition to cutting energy costs in transportation. It takes much less energy to keep food frozen than it takes to

SNAPSHOTS **BING WRIGHT**

"Once you've tried fresh tomatoes, you'll

Catskill Mountains, New York
Gardener

In the Catskill Mountains, where frost in May and September is not unusual, Bing Wright grows bushels of tomatoes. He plants about 50 tomato plants, he figures, in a garden maybe 20 by 30 feet in size. From that small plot, he can harvest enough tomatoes to enjoy all year long.

It's incredibly simple to make a lot of tomato products, he says. Plant a variety of tomatoes. When they are ripe, red, and ready to fall from the vine, you simply wash them, cut them in half (removing any bad parts), and then strain them. He uses a Squeezo Strainer (made by Best Products), which traps the skin and the seeds and lets the puree pass through for you to use right away in a sauce, soup, or salsa, or to store for another day. No cooking is necessary.

Bing stores the puree in quart-sized containers—approximately three cups

ship food hundreds, even thousands, of miles and keep it fresh along the way. Dried and canned foods can also be nutritious options.

FIND LOCAL PROCESSORS The key to eating food that has been preserved in some way for the winter months is to buy it from local processors. Most frozen or canned packaged food will name the processor and distributor on the package. Let that address be your guide to help you determine if it is local or not. Most food is frozen on the West Coast because of the longer growing season. Food is frozen immediately in local processing plants after being picked, to retain the most nutritive qualities. East Coast food processors do exist, however, and once you identify a local brand, look for it whenever you shop.

For help locating food processors near you, contact the American Frozen Food Institute, 2000 Corporate Ridge, Suite 1000, McLean, VA 22102.

never go back. ”

per container, enough for a meal for a family of four—in a large freezer. On average, he puts aside 40 or so containers per year, keeping his family in fresh tomatoes from September to May.

Bing Wright will often make a cold sauce with his stored tomatoes by mixing 3 cups of puree with olive oil and garlic to go on pasta or fish, or in a chopped salad. Heating the puree into a warm sauce is also fast and easy: A sauce made from fresh ingredients takes about 20 minutes—and tastes delicious.

At the end of the season, to ripen tomatoes that otherwise won't ripen on the vine when cooler temperatures arrive, Bing suggests this reliable technique: Lay the green tomatoes on a newspaper in a cool, dark place like the basement. They should ripen in a week or so. Eat when ripe or turn into puree for freezing. It's that simple!

Preserving the Harvest

While it isn't difficult to buy local, and even organic, produce during harvest time, it can be difficult and expensive to maintain a diet of those foods in the winter and early spring. On the other hand, after savoring the flavors of fresh foods and enjoying their environmental and health benefits, it can be frustrating to switch back to lackluster supermarket produce. One viable way of solving this problem is to preserve local food while it is still in season. Food preservation is perhaps the most useful tool for establishing a green kitchen year-round, and the rewards are immense. Opening a jar of dried tomatoes to add to pasta in the middle of a January snowstorm, or spreading your own strawberry jam on toast for your children for a February breakfast, is very satisfying. It is a treat in the winter to know where your food came from.

For the most part, the days of preserving food by standing over a hot stove canning for two weeks straight during the dog days of August are long gone. Most people today approach preserving food in an eclectic way, according to taste and time. A popular combination

Do your best to find eggs, dairy, meat, and game from local sources as well. Check at your farmers' market, or go to www.eatwellguide.com to find suppliers nearest you.

Simple Stewardship

TRUE FOOD MEANS A SENSE OF PLACE

Being connected to your community is a mainstay of psychological health. What better way to connect than through food? Really knowing local maple syrup if you live in New England is a matter of pride, as is really knowing a good gumbo in the Gulf South, or wild rice in the Great Lakes areas. Place-based food traditions celebrate diversity and community, while exploring the natural and cultural history of the region. Saving endangered culinary cultures also helps save indigenous plants and animals.

Food Safety Rules of Thumb

	MICROORGANISMS (MAY CAUSE ILLNESS)	**ENZYMES (MAY SPOIL FOOD)**
Heat	Halted below 32°F Retarded at 32-50°F Thrive at 50-120°F Killed at 212-240°F in high-acid foods Killed at 240°F in low-acid foods	Slowed but not halted below 32°F Slowed at 32-50°F Thrive in 85-120°F Inactivated at 240°F
Moisture	Halted when below 35 percent Thrive when damp Retarded when saturated	No effect
Acidity	Hostile environment	Slows process
Sugar	Hostile environment	Variable
Salt	Hostile environment	Variable
Oxygen	Most thrive in air *C. botulinum* grows with no oxygen	No effect

of techniques people tend to use includes freezing most fruit, vegetables, and ready-made foods like tomato sauces; drying fruit for children's snacks, and tomatoes and vegetables for winter soups; pickling cucumbers; preserving berries; canning tomatoes (it takes one full day to can 50 quarts of tomatoes); and, if there is space, using cold storage for root vegetables. The popularity of this combination of preserving techniques is not surprising: It is manageable, even for those with very busy lives, and it keeps food preservation interesting.

STOPPING THE GROWTH OF MICROORGANISMS When produce is picked, microorganisms—bacteria, yeast, and molds—slowly but surely start growing on it. They can ultimately make the food inedible and sometimes even poisonous. But microorganisms are all affected by heat, oxygen, moisture, and acid content. Each preserving technique manipulates these elements, and thereby the microorganisms, in a different way.

Canning, for example, heats the food to such a high temperature that the microorganisms are killed. The reason that high-heat processing is so important for canning is that some bacteria—like *Clostridium botulinum*, a form of botulism—thrive in an oxygen-free environment, as is found inside a jar of canned vegetables. The jar needs to be heated to a temperature high enough to kill *C. botulinum* (240°F). Freezing, on the other hand, reduces the temperature to such a degree that the multiplication of microorganisms is halted. Microorganisms also depend on moisture. Drying sucks the moisture out of the food so that microorganisms can't grow, but it isn't as successful as freezing for halting microorganisms, as anyone with mold allergies can testify. Microorganisms do not thrive in acidic, salty, or high-sugar environments, either, which is why all these techniques of pickling represent another successful, and time-honored, preservation technique.

If you live at a high altitude (more than 5,000 feet above sea level), find out more about canning in your region. Call your county's cooperative extension service, federally funded offices administered by state agricultural colleges, and ask for guidelines for home preserving at your altitude.

STOPPING THE ENZYME PROCESS Enzymes cause chemical transformations that ripen fruit and vegetables. They also continue beyond ripening, causing produce to decay. This natural process needs to be halted in food you want to preserve. High heat, freezing temperatures, or a highly acidic environment can halt enzyme activity.

Time is an important factor. The sooner a food is processed after being picked, the better. Food that is cut open has to be tended to immediately. The sooner vegetables are plunged into a blanching hot-water or steam bath, for example, or the sooner fruit is treated with ascorbic acid or citric acid, the less enzyme damage

Preservation Techniques

TECHNIQUE	HOW IT WORKS
Freezing	Cold stops enzyme process and growth of microorganisms; food is stored in airtight containers.
Drying	Food is heated, and drying process removes moisture from it.
Root Cellars	Root cellars maintain a constant temperature of 32–35°F for most foods, 50–60°F for others. Root cellar storage slows enzyme process and microorganism growth.
Canning	Glass jars containing food are treated in a boiling water bath. Oxygen is removed from inside the jars and the food is processed at a high heat. The food must be acidic.
Pressure Canning	As with canning, high heat affects glass jars containing food; oxygen is removed and the food is processed.
Jams and Jellies	Oxygen is removed; the food is made acidic as needed, sweetened, and processed at high heat.
Pickling	Usually oxygen is removed; the food has a high acid content; it is usually processed at a high heat.
Smoking*	Salt reduces growth of bacteria and pulls out moisture; sugar curing reduces growth of bacteria; smoke coats the meat, protecting it from rancidity; the food is dried, removing moisture.
Curing*	Salt and sugar both reduce growth of bacteria; salt pulls out moisture; the food is dried.

*Due to the high salt content of curing and smoking and the health concerns of by-products of smoke, these processes are not recommended as a healthful means of food preservation.

your food will have. Enzymes work at different speeds for different fruit and vegetables. A cool root cellar halts enzymes just enough to keep a potato for a number of months, but a strawberry would hardly last a few days and needs to be frozen or canned.

General Guidelines for Preserving Food

The three rules of thumb for preserving food are to be scrupulously clean, to follow directions to a T, and to work fast (except for preparing food for root

Shopping & Saving

WHEN FACED WITH CHOICES...

Some simple guidelines to help prioritize:

If you can't buy locally produced food, then **buy organic.** This is one of the most readily available alternatives in the market. Making this choice protects the environment and also protects your body from harsh chemicals and hormones.

If you can't buy organic food, then **buy from a family farm.** When faced with a variety of cheeses made by Kraft or by Cabot, choose Cabot, a dairy co-op in Vermont, as the better choice. Supporting family farms helps to keep food processing decisions out of the hands of the corporate conglomeration.

If you can't buy food from a family farm, then **buy from a local business.** Basics like coffee and bread make buying locally difficult. Try a local coffee shop or bakery to keep your food dollar close to home.

If you can't buy food from a local business, then **buy for *terroir*,** a French word suggesting the taste of the earth. Purchase foods famous for the region they are grown in and support the agriculture that produces your favorite nonlocal foods such as Brie cheese from Brie, France, or Parmesan cheese from Parma, Italy.

Thanks to Jessica Prentice, Locavores.com, and to the Buy Local Challenge, BuyLocalChallenge.org, for these rules.

cellars). Contaminated food is no joke. Nor is food that has lost all its nutritive value because of improper handling. While canning involves the greatest danger of deadly food poisoning if done improperly, all techniques must be approached responsibly. This being said, you should not be frightened away from "putting food by," as experienced preservers like to say. Fortunately, if the rules of food preservation are followed, you should be guaranteed excellent, flavorful, healthful—and pleasingly local—results.

Pretreating Before Preserving

Most fruit and vegetables should be pretreated before drying, freezing, or canning, to halt the enzyme action and the early growth of microorganisms. One way to do it is to blanch the food. Blanching heats water or steam to 212°F, the temperature needed to stop enzyme activity in acidic foods. Blanching is also recommended for most vegetables that are to be dried and canned. Fruit is typically pretreated using acids such as ascorbic acid (vitamin C) or citric acid to stop the enzyme process from browning the fruit once it has been cut.

Foods being canned must be heated to 240°F for the appropriate amount of time to kill the deadly *C. botulinum.* See the time chart on pages 27-28.

ALL ABOUT BLANCHING Blanching partially precooks vegetables by scalding them in boiling water or steam. It halts the enzyme process and helps maintain the flavor of the vegetables.

There are two kinds of blanching—water blanching and steam blanching. With water blanching, food is plunged into rapidly boiling water so it is completely covered. With steam blanching, the food sits in steam produced by water boiling under it. Steaming retains the most nutritive value in the food, but some foods, such as greens, mat together when steamed, so they need to be water-blanched.

Ironically, if food is not blanched long enough, enzyme activity will speed up. Overblanching, on the other hand, robs food of some nutrient value as well as color, crispness, and flavor.

WATER BLANCHING

Equipment you will need:

A large stainless steel or enamel pot with a tight-fitting cover, capable of holding two or more gallons of rapidly boiling water

Cutting board, sharp knife, and vegetable peeler

Wire basket or strainer insert that fits inside the pot (preferably two: one for ice bath, if freezing, and one for the boiling water bath)

Sink or large bowl, very clean, and capable of holding ice and water in quantity greater than in pot

- Clean your equipment carefully: cutting boards, knives, pot, sink, strainers, and any items necessary for canning, freezing, or drying.
- Fill the pot with water (about one gallon per pound of vegetables). Insert basket/strainer and heat to a rolling boil.
- If you plan on freezing the vegetables, prepare an ice water bath. Empty at least two trays of ice cubes per pound of vegetables into a sink or large bowl.
- While water is heating, prepare produce by washing, trimming off stems, coring and slicing when appropriate, and cutting off bad spots.
- Keeping the water at a full boil, pull out the basket or strainer, fill it with vegetables (all one type), plunge them into the boiling water, and quickly cover the pot to maintain a rolling boil.
- Immediately set the timer for the appropriate number of minutes needed to blanch the particular vegetable you are processing. Food blanched too long becomes food boiled, and it loses crispness and nutrients.

If you do not have a wire basket or strainer for water blanching, cheesecloth will do, but it does not allow as much water to circulate among the vegetables.

Blanching Time for Vegetables

VEGETABLE	BLANCHING TIME (IN MINUTES)
Artichokes, trimmed	4, small to medium (add juice of one lemon to blanching water)
Asparagus	2-4, depending on size
Beans (green)	3-4, depending on size
Beans (lima)	3-4, depending on size
Beets, sliced	Simmer until tender
Beet greens	2 (water blanch only)
Broccoli florets	2-4, depending on size
Brussels sprouts	3-5, depending on size
Cabbage wedges	3
Carrots	3-4, whole
Cauliflower florets	3-5, depending on size (add juice of one lemon to blanching water)
Celery	3
Collard greens	3 (water blanch only)
Corn on the cob	5-7, depending on size
Corn, cut kernels	6-8
Cucumber slices	none; instead, puree for freezing
Eggplant slices	4
Greens	3 (water blanch only)
Herbs	1
Kale	1 (water blanch only)
Kohlrabi	2 (small, whole), 1 (sliced)
Leek	no need to blanch before freezing

VEGETABLE	BLANCHING TIME (IN MINUTES)
Mushrooms, slices	2-4 (add juice of one lemon to blanching water)
Okra, unsliced	2-4 (add juice of one lemon to blanching water)
Onions	no need to blanch before freezing
Parsley	15-20 seconds
Parsnips, sliced	2
Peas, shelled	1
Peppers (green, red)	3 (halve to freeze)
Peppers (hot)	no need to blanch before freezing
Potatoes	bake or fry before freezing
Pumpkin, cubed	bake before freezing
Rutabagas, sliced	2
Spinach	2 (water blanch only)
Squash, summer, sliced	3
Squash, winter	bake before freezing
Sweet potatoes	bake thoroughly; dip in mild lemon juice solution beforehand
Swiss chard	2 (water blanch only)
Tomatoes	boil until skins crack; cool and remove skins; simmer 10 minutes
Turnips, sliced	2

- When time is up, pull the vegetables out of the boiling water and plunge them immediately into the ice water bath.
- Once the vegetables are completely cold, process further to store them by freezing or canning.

STEAM BLANCHING

Equipment you will need:

A large stainless steel or enamel pot with a tight-fitting cover, capable of holding two or more gallons of rapidly boiling water

Cutting board, sharp knife, and vegetable peeler

A steamer tray that fits into your large pot

Wire basket or strainer insert that fits inside the pot (preferably two: one for ice bath, if freezing, and one for the boiling water bath)

- Follow the procedures for water blanching, but instead of filling the pot with water, place the steamer inside the pot and fill the pot with enough water to just cover the steamer. Once the steam starts escaping, place one layer of vegetables at a time on the steamer tray, covering the pot as you prepare each layer and making sure that the water does not boil away.

A steamer tray is a metal basket with feet that fits inside a cooking pot. The feet hold it up above the boiling water, and it cradles the vegetables so that they are cooked by steam without touching the boiling water. Steaming keeps more vitamins in cooked vegetables.

GIVING FRUIT THE ACID TREATMENT When you squeeze lemon juice onto a freshly cut avocado or apple to keep it from browning, you are giving the fruit an acid treatment. Acid treatments reduce enzyme activity and create a hostile environment for microorganisms; they are used for freezing, drying, and canning many fruits, and also for some vegetables.

Equipment you will need:

Stainless steel or enamel pans or bowls

Ascorbic acid, available in health food stores

Slotted spoon

Baking sheets

Add acid to apples, avocados, bananas, cherries, mangoes, melons, nectarines, peaches, pears, and persimmons as you process them to preserve them.

Bottled lemon juice is recommended for increasing acidity instead of freshly squeezed lemon juice, because the bottled version has a consistent acidity.

- Place 2 quarts of cold water and 3 or 4 ice cubes in pan or bowl.
- Add 3 tablespoons lemon juice.
- Add fruit (loosely packed, not crushed) to pan or bowl.
- Leave in pan from 1 to 5 minutes.
- Remove fruit with slotted spoon, and spread out on clean baking sheets to air-dry.

Freezing

Food preserved by freezing loses fewer vitamins and minerals in processing than it does when preserved by any other method. The faster it is frozen, the more nutrients it retains. Freezing is also the quickest, easiest, and safest procedure of all the techniques for preserving food. Vegetables are simply blanched, cooled, packaged, and

Shopping & Saving

WHAT'S BEST TO FREEZE FOOD IN?

Canning jars made of tempered glass are just the thing for freezing. They come in pint and quart sizes and are available in most hardware stores. Tempered glass has been put through extreme heating and cooling during its manufacture, so it is five to six times stronger than regular glass. Nevertheless, all food in glass jars should be cooled before being placed in the freezer.

The only other reliable and accessible freezer packaging is heavy plastic—which presents a dilemma. Plastic food containers are undesirable not only because their use depletes virgin resources, but also because the chemicals in plastic can migrate into warm and fatty foods, a potential health hazard. See more on plastic food containers in Step 8, pages 308-313.

frozen. Fruit is cut, dipped in an ascorbic acid bath, and frozen, or cooked in a syrup and frozen. Tomato sauces can be made when tomatoes are falling off the vines, then frozen for a ready-made midwinter spaghetti sauce. Lasagna can be made in double batches and frozen for a busy day. By placing food into temperatures of around 0°F, as is found in most freezers, one can ensure that the activity of microorganisms is halted and the enzyme process is significantly slowed.

SECRETS FOR SUCCESSFUL FREEZING Freezer burn is the common term used to describe food that has dried out after it has been frozen. It tastes like cardboard at best. You need to package the food you are going to place in the freezer in containers that hold in all the moisture. Any food in a package that is not sealed properly—aluminum foil with a tear, a freezer bag that isn't closed, and even a freezer bag with a lot of empty space in it—and any food wrapped in packaging without a tight vapor barrier will experience freezer burn. Plastic freezer bags, rigid plastic freezer containers, and glass canning jars all provide a vapor barrier and are airtight.

Enzymes and microorganisms will continue doing their work until the food is placed in the deep cold of a freezer, so freezing food fast is important. Plan ahead so that you have enough time to completely process and cool the food; don't leave it to sit overnight, even in the refrigerator. You also need to make sure the freezer maintains its 0°F temperature for a quick freeze. If you add too much food

Want to freeze your broccoli in separate florets so you can take out a few at a time? Blanch the florets, then arrange them on a cookie sheet to cool, laying them out so the pieces don't touch one another. Freeze them this way for three to four hours, then repackage the florets in one container. Now they won't stick together.

We should be producing the fullest variety of foods to be consumed locally, in the countryside itself and in nearby towns and cities: meats, grains, table vegetables, fruits and nuts, dairy products, poultry, and eggs.

—WENDELL BERRY, FARMER AND POET

to the freezer all at once, it will have a hard time maintaining that temperature. The general rule of thumb is to add food to a freezer no faster than one pound per cubic foot of freezer space a day.

CHOOSING A FREEZER If you plan to freeze a substantial amount of food, there is no getting around the need for a large-capacity freezer. This one requirement can be an expensive one, but not as expensive as you might think. At the time of the writing of this book, Sears was selling a 7.5-cubic-foot upright freezer for $300 and a 7.2-cubic-foot chest freezer for $200. You can pack a lot of food into freezers this size. The advantage of buying a new freezer is that you will benefit from the advances in energy efficiency. Older freezers will cost more to run, but you will pay much less up front. Used large-capacity freezers are available for as little as $50.

Wide-mouth jars are often handier to use because you can fill and empty them more easily. They are ideal for homemade sauces such as apple and tomato.

Foods Good for Freezing

The sky's the limit when it comes to foods that are good candidates for freezing. In fact, the only limit, really, is your imagination. Not quite everything freezes well—lettuce is out, cucumbers need to be made into a soup,

Freezable Fruit & Vegetables

Fruit	Vegetables
Apples, apricots, avocados, berries, cherries, coconut, currants, figs, grapefruit and oranges, grapes, melons, nectarines, peaches, pears, persimmons, pineapple, plums, prunes, rhubarb, watermelons	Artichokes, asparagus, beans, beets, broccoli, Brussels sprouts, cabbage, carrots, cauliflower, celery, collards, corn, eggplant, greens, herbs, kohlrabi, leeks, onions, okra, parsnips, peas, peppers, potatoes, pumpkins, rutabagas, soybeans, squash (summer and winter), sweet potatoes, tomatoes, turnips

and beans can get mealy—but you may be surprised at the variety of foods suitable for freezing. Buying eggs on sale can be worth it, for example, because they freeze beautifully—crack a bunch, blend with a fork, and pour into ice cube trays. Once frozen, place individual "egg cubes" in a freezer bag for future use. One cube equals one egg. Even dairy products like milk, cream, cottage cheese, and butter can be frozen! Buy food when it is cheap and locally produced, and freeze it for later use.

As soon as you can after the produce enters your kitchen, prepare it for freezing. Wash, peel, slice, core, and cut away bad spots.

FREEZING VEGETABLES Most vegetables need to be blanched (briefly cooked) before freezing.

- Use a double sink or a sink and a large pan. Scrub them until they are scrupulously clean, and then rinse them thoroughly.
- While the vegetables are blanching, fill one sink or the pan with cold water and ice from two or three ice trays.
- Once the vegetables have been blanched the correct amount of time, plunge them, basket and all, into the ice-cold water.
- Cool the vegetables thoroughly in the ice water, and then with a slotted spoon remove them and place them on a cookie sheet so the pieces aren't touching each other.
- Place immediately in the freezer for three to four hours. Remove and drop into freezer bags or freezer containers, label, and return to the freezer.

Label all containers of frozen food with a grease pencil. Avoid permanent ink markers: Their solvents linger in the environment and can be toxic, and an indelible label can be annoying when you want to reuse the container.

FREEZING FRUIT IN SYRUP Fruit is usually frozen in a surrounding syrup, but it doesn't have to be supersweet. Here are a few formulas for fruit-freezing syrups:

- ½ cup honey to 4 cups water
- 1 cup sugar or unrefined sugar to 4 cups water
- ½ cup maple syrup to 4 cups water

You can also make an all-fruit syrup by putting the fruit in a pan, pouring in fruit juice enough to cover it, and simmering the mixture until the fruit is cooked. Freeze the fruit and its juice-based syrup together. You can also freeze juice and fruit together without cooking.

Other Reasons for Freezing

Freezing food is a great way to establish a healthful diet in our very busy lives. Food can be frozen in advance for days when you know you won't have time to cook. Whenever you find that you have the time and desire to cook, make extra of everything and freeze it. That way, you have home-cooked food made with love even when you don't have the time to cook it.

Make "herb cubes" by cutting up some fresh herbs, placing a teaspoon or so of them in an ice cube tray, covering them with water, and freezing. Make mint cubes for your tea in the winter or basil cubes for your vegetable soup.

- If you enjoy making soup in the winter, keep a large freezer bag of loose vegetables stored in the freezer. Every time you are chopping vegetables, cut a little extra and throw them into this all-purpose "soup bag."
- If you like pesto, make several batches at once. Spoon into meal-size yogurt containers, and freeze. (Omit the pine nuts when you do this, and add just before serving.)
- If you don't use up gingerroot very quickly, and tend to throw a lot away because it goes bad, freeze some root

Shopping & Saving

FREEZER ECONOMIES

The freezer is the perfect aid for practicing thrift. Not only can you buy food when it is cheap and freeze it, but you can also significantly reduce the amount of food you waste. For example, if bananas are beginning to get overripe and you don't have time to make banana bread, simply mash up the bananas, add a little lemon juice, and freeze them until you have time to bake.

in a small freezer bag, take it out, and grate off only as much as you need, then replace the root in the freezer.

Freezing Rules of Thumb

- Never pack a canning jar, freezer container, or freezer bag completely full. Water expands when it freezes. A plastic bag can explode and a canning jar can crack in the freezer.
- Make sure that containers are sealed completely before freezing! This can make the difference between delicious and tasteless food.
- Label and date all food that is put in the freezer.
- As a general guideline, don't refreeze food that has been thawed, especially meat and seafood. Refrozen food loses its flavor and texture, and the food may have become slightly spoiled when it thawed.
- Most produce lasts up to ten months in a freezer.

Drying Food

The increasing popularity of sun-dried tomatoes has generated interest in drying other foods at home. Drying concentrates the flavors of foods, making them welcome additions to many dishes.

Moisture is an essential ingredient needed by microorganisms to multiply, and by drying food—removing the moisture in it—you retard the growth of those microorganisms. Once the food is dry, it is very lightweight, ideal for camping or travel. Stored in airtight containers, it will last a long time. Dried vegetables are excellent for soups (peas, zucchinis, carrots, string beans, tomatoes). Dried fruit makes a good snack and can be rehydrated for use in pies and other desserts.

If you live in a climate that is sunny, warm, and dry, you need little more than a drying rack or two to place in the sun. It doesn't get much easier or cheaper than that!

A friend has a few pear trees and gives me bagfuls of pears in October. I line them up in windowsills until they are perfectly ripe, and then I take a few evenings to freeze them, by cutting them into slices, coring them, and cooking with water, honey to taste, and freshly grated gingerroot. I cool the mixture, package it in quart freezer containers (meal-size), and freeze them. I could add a bit of lemon juice to make sure the pears don't brown, but I find I don't need to.–*A.B.B.*

On the other hand, if your climate is more humid and you want to do a lot of drying, dehydrating equipment is essential. But maybe you want to start off slowly and experiment with simply drying some tomatoes.

Three Secrets of Food Drying Success

The three main elements necessary for drying food successfully are heat, time, and air circulation.

HEAT The USDA recommends a steady heat of 140°F for drying food. While this is a little higher than some books recommend, mold growth is inhibited at 140°F, an important factor.

TIME Give the drying process the time it needs. Interrupting it could encourage mold growth. If you have an electric food dehydrator, keep the dehydrator going continuously until the food is dried. The faster food is dried, the more nutrients it maintains.

AIR CIRCULATION When food dries, moisture is pulled to the food's surface, where it evaporates. When surrounding air doesn't circulate—in a fanless electric dehydrator or in the oven with the door closed—moisture clings to the surface and mold grows.

To avoid having all of your pans end up in the freezer, buy inexpensive, reusable aluminum pans, available in most supermarkets. Make double batches of casseroles, lasagna, and favorite dishes, transfer them to the aluminum pans, and freeze.

DRYING EQUIPMENT To dry food, you can make your own racks and dryer, buy dryers including racks, or use your oven—carefully. To make your own drying racks, stretch cheesecloth or stainless steel screening over a wooden frame and nail or staple securely. Commercially available food dehydrators come shaped like a box or a round tower, with trays, heating coils, and sometimes a fan. Make sure that the dehydrator has adequate ventilation.

You can dry food in your oven, but you have to be sure not to cook the food. Crack open the oven door for air

Drying Fruit and Vegetables

FRUIT/VEGGIE	PRETREATMENT	CUT	DRY TIME (IN HRS.)	WHEN DONE
Apples	ascorbic acid	slice	6	suedelike
Asparagus	steam blanch	1-inch slices	2-3	leathery
Bananas	none	slice	2-6	brittle
Beans, green	steam blanch	whole/sliced	3-5	brittle
Berries	none	whole	4	like raisins
Broccoli	steam blanch	florets	3-6	brittle
Carrots	steam blanch	slice	3-5	suedelike
Cauliflower	steam blanch	florets	3-6	brittle
Cherries	prick skin	pitted	6	like raisins
Celery	steam blanch	1-inch slices	2-4	brittle
Corn on cob	steam blanch	whole	2-6	brittle
Corn off cob	steam on cob	cut off cob	1-3	brittle
Grapes	none	halve/whole	8	like raisins
Mushrooms	none	slice	4-5	suedelike
Onions	none	dice	1-6	brittle
Peaches	ascorbic acid	slice	6	suedelike
Pears	ascorbic acid	slice	6	suedelike
Peas	steam blanch	shell/whole pod	3-4	dry/brittle
Peppers	none	sliced	3-5	brittle
Potatoes	steam blanch	slice	2-6	brittle
Pumpkins	steam blanch	slice	4-6	brittle
Spinach	steam blanch	destemmed	2-5	brittle
Sweet potatoes	steam blanch	slice	3-6	suedelike/ brittle
Tomatoes	none	slice	4-8	suedelike
Zucchini	steam blanch	slice	2-5	brittle

*Dry Time is equal to the number of hours in the oven or dehydrator, not in the sun. Double the time for sun drying (not including night hours).

circulation. Also, only use the oven if you can ensure a temperature of around 140°F, no higher. Often a gas stove with a pilot light is enough; set an electric oven at the lowest possible setting.

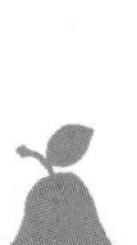

Drying sheds are fine if you live in a very dry climate, such as the Southwest, but most outdoor sheds are not very effective for drying foods because the nights are so damp and dewy that the moisture seeps in and interferes with the drying process.

General Drying Procedure

- Wash, core, and remove stems of ripe fruit or vegetables to be dried.
- Cut the produce into uniform, thin slices. This is important, as thicker sections take longer to dry than others, overdrying some parts and underdrying others.
- Blanch vegetables or acid-treat fruit, as described earlier in this chapter.
- Place fruits and vegetables on dryer trays. Lay them in one layer, without overlapping.
- Start the drying process, be it in the sun, oven, or an electric food dehydrator.
- If you are using a solar drying method, remember to bring the food in before dusk and place in a warm oven—lowest setting possible—for the night.

Fun, Kids, Pleasure

MAKING FRUIT LEATHERS

Fruit leathers, popular with children, can be made at home—more local, more organic, more fun!

1. Wash, core, and remove the stems of ripe fruit.
2. In a food processor, puree the fruit until it forms a thick paste.
3. Using a spatula, smooth the paste onto an oiled cookie sheet.
4. Dry in the oven at the lowest temperature setting or in a dehydrator until it is no longer sticky.

Know Your Acid Levels

Low-Acid Foods (pH > 4.6)	High-Acid Foods (pH < 4.6)
Pumpkins, carrots, beets, squash, beans, spinach, cabbage, turnips, peppers, sweet potatoes, asparagus, potatoes, mushrooms, peas, corn	Citrus fruit, plums, apples, strawberries, rhubarb, berries, cherries, peaches, apricots, pears, pineapple
Required Equipment: Pressure canner only	**Required Equipment:** Boiling water canner or pressure canner

- Consult the table for drying times and adjust the drying time to your taste.
- Discard any dried food that appears moldy. Most dried food lasts for six to nine months.

Canning Food

Canning works to preserve food by deactivating enzymes and killing microorganisms. It requires heating the foods to a very high heat for a specific length of time. Once canned at the right temperature, the food remains in containers that are airtight, ensuring no further contamination.

To can food, you must determine if it is low-acid or high-acid. Any food with a pH of 4.6 or below (high-acid) must be heated to a temperature of 212°F in a boiling water canner for a length of time specific to that food. Any food with a pH above 4.6 (low-acid foods) must be heated to a temperature of 240°F, and only in a pressure canner. Some tomatoes fall in the middle, especially the new low-acid varieties (see page 41).

We don't advise buying food dehydrators without fans, as the food can more easily get moldy and spoiled.

Who determines, and for what strange reasons, the social status of a vegetable? —M. F. K. FISHER, *SERVE IT FORTH*

BANNING BOTULISM Some people are wary of canning for fear of the deadly *C. botulinum*, a bacterium that grows in canned foods and causes botulism, which is often fatal. The bacterium grows in soil, so it is commonly found on plants. It becomes a deadly poison as it develops spores, which carry the botulism. The bacterium thrives in the exact conditions found inside a container of canned food: room temperature, no oxygen, and a lot of moisture. *C. botulinum* has no smell and does not indicate its presence in any way. It is killed at high heat: 240°F. Canning directions are designed precisely to kill *C. botulinum*, so if you follow every procedure exactly, there should be no risk.

Canning Equipment

Pint and quart canning jars, lids, and rubber rings (for certain types of jar)

Spoons, ladles, slotted spoons, colander

Knives, vegetable peelers, corers, etc.

Funnels

Jar gripper

Kitchen timer

TRUE TIP

Stainless steel screening is expensive and hard to find, but it is well worth the money and effort. Try finding it online from McMasters-Carr: *www.mcmaster.com.*

CHOOSE YOUR CANNER Boiling water canners are usually enamel and come with a wire rack insert to hold the jars in place and a cover. The canner needs to be deep enough for rapidly boiling water to completely cover quart jars. (When you are in the store to buy a boiling water canner, it is worth placing a quart jar in the canner to make sure there is enough headroom.)

No matter what kind of food you are canning, high-or low-acid, it is packed either hot or cold in jars, and in a liquid. These two choices are called either "hot packs"—the food is placed in the jars cooked and hot, and hot juice, water, or a syrup is poured over it—or "raw packs"—the food is placed in the canning jar without being cooked and is covered with boiling juice or water.

If you cook a food for canning, don't let it cool before you pack it into the jars.

PREP STEPS FOR CANNING It is critically important that your cutting board, sink, and all equipment be scrupulously clean. Make sure that jars and canners are in perfect working order. Wash lids and rings according to manufacturer's instructions. The two-piece lids are recommended for ease of use and because they are designed to create an airtight seal. Sterilize the jars and a metal knife by placing them in a large container with enough water to cover, bringing to a hard boil, and boiling for 15 minutes. Leave jars in the hot water until ready to fill. (If you add hot food to cold jars, the jars can crack.) Work as fast as you can. The faster the process is completed, the less chance of any new contamination with microorganisms.

Do not confuse a pressure canner with a pressure cooker. Pressure canners are especially made for processing foods with steam and are equipped with a safety valve and a petcock opening. Fortunately, pressure canners are coming back into popularity and are easier to find than they were even ten years ago.

FOR FRUIT & PICKLES IN A BOILING WATER CANNER Fill the boiling water canner with enough water to clear the tops of the jars by at least one inch. Turn the heat on

Cooking & Eating

TOMATOES: A SPECIAL CASE FOR CANNING

In general, tomatoes are high-acid foods, but not all tomatoes have a pH below 4.6. In recent years low-acid varieties have been developed that can push the pH above 4.6, into the low-acid category. The best rule of thumb is to increase the acid content of any tomatoes you plan to process in a boiling water canner. The Cornell Cooperative Extension Service recommends adding 2 tablespoons of bottled lemon juice per quart of tomatoes. You can pressure-can them without extra acid.

high; heat to 180°F. Wash produce thoroughly. Peel, core, slice, or otherwise prepare the food for canning. Treat apples, cherries, peaches, or pears with acid treatment as described earlier in this chapter. Let them soak for ten minutes. Remove with a slotted spoon. Have a kettle on the stove ready with boiling water to replenish the water in the pan when needed. If you add cold water, the jars will crack.

Variations on Packing Liquids

You will need up to a cup of liquid to pack a quart jar. For fruit, you can use water, juice, or a sweet syrup.

WATER Bring to a boil before packing.

You must use new rings and lids every time you can. Used rings may have lost their ability to make a perfect seal. Also, you must use jars designed for canning, so that the glass can withstand the high heat.

JUICE If the fruit is juicy and being hot-packed, you may get enough juice from the cooking process, with maybe the addition of a little water, to cover the fruit once it is packed in the jars. If not, use store-bought juice diluted to taste (a lot of varieties of juice are available), or make your own by simmering fruit with a small amount of water, straining off the fruit when soft and mushy, and packing with the liquid. Before packing, heat juice just to boiling.

SYRUP Heavy syrups have a one-to-one ratio between sweetener and liquid. Avoid those, and make thin syrups with whole-food sweeteners like honey or sorghum molasses instead of refined white sugar. The basic formula for a light syrup for canning is to combine 1 cup sugar with 3 cups of a water and fruit juice combination. Slowly bring to a boil. Simmer at a low boil for six minutes, stirring constantly. For a lighter syrup, add up to 6 cups water or fruit juice.

Packing and Processing into Canning Jars

- Using slotted spoons, ladles, funnels, or whatever works best, fill the sterilized jars with fruit or pickles. Hot packs should be packed loosely; raw packs can be packed tighter. Pour the liquid over the food, leaving the right amount of headroom.

- Slide a sterilized knife around the inside edge of the jars to remove any air pockets. With a clean cloth, wipe the tops of the jars to make sure there is no food that could interfere with a perfect seal. Screw the tops on the jars securely.

Ba's Bread and Butter Pickles

Pickles and relish require more elaborate preparation than do fruit and vegetables. Multiple fresh ingredients are chopped and added together, sometimes to sit overnight, and then heated with spices for flavoring. Here, from Annie's sister, is one of our favorite recipes for transforming cucumbers to canned pickles for winter. MAKES 4 QUARTS

- 6 quarts thin, horizontally sliced pickling cucumbers
- 6 medium onions, thinly sliced
- ½ cup pickling salt
- ice cubes
- 1½ quarts white vinegar
- 4 cups unrefined sugar
- ½ cup whole mustard seeds
- 1 tablespoon celery seed
- 2 tablespoons pickling spice, wrapped and tied in cheesecloth
- 8 pint jars or 4 quart jars

1. Put the cucumbers, onions, and salt in a large enamel pot. Stir to combine well. Cover with ice and let mixture sit overnight.

2. Drain the contents of the pot into a colander and rinse well with several changes of water.

3. In a large enamel or stainless steel pot, combine the vinegar, sugar, mustard seeds, celery seed, and pickling spice. Bring the mixture to a boil for several minutes and then add the cucumber and onion mixture. Bring just to a low boil and pack in sterilized jars.

4. Process in a boiling water bath (15 minutes for pints, 20 minutes for quarts) with 1 inch of water covering the tops of the jars.

If you live at a high altitude, add more time for the boiling water bath during canning.

- Place the jars in the canner, making sure they are covered by at least one inch of water. Replace the lid.
- Bring the water to a hard boil. Start timing once it is boiling. Add hot water if needed to cover the jars.
- When time is up, remove the jars and place them on racks. Then seal, if the directions for your type of lid require it.
- Let the jars cool (up to 12 hours or even more). Do not retighten lids! If any seals are loose, discard or reprocess from the beginning. After the jars have cooled, test the seal according to manufacturer's instructions. Label jars with date and contents.

Pressure Canning

Many of the rules for boiling water canning apply for pressure canning too.

- Pour 2 or 3 inches of hot water into the pressure canner. Place the jars on the rack. Close the cover of the canner completely. At this time leave the gauge open and do not close the petcock.
- Heat until steam escapes, then time for 10 minutes. (This is preparing the steamer for canning; it is not canning time.) Follow manufacturer's directions for setting the pressure to 10 pounds (240°F).
- Start timing once 10 pounds has been reached.
- Take the canner off the heat, return pressure to zero, and wait before opening, according to the manufacturer's instructions.

There are no simple answers to preserving farms and agriculture, but so far, farmers' markets have been the most incredible solution going.

—ELIZABETH RYAN, ORCHARDIST, BREEZY HILL ORCHARDS, STAATSBURG, N.Y.

Canning Acid Foods in a Boiling Water Bath

FOOD	PREP FOR CANNING	HOT PACK=HP RAW PACK=RP	HEADROOM (between lid and top of food)	TIME IN BOILING WATER (in minutes)
Apples	Slice	HP	½ inch	Pint jars: 15 Quart jars: 20
Apricots	Peel, halve, pit	HP	½ inch	Pint jars: 20 Quart jars: 25
Berries		HP or RP	½ inch	Pint jars: 10 Quart jars: 15
Cherries	Prick or pit	HP or RP	½ inch	Pint jars: 25 Quart jars: 25
Grapefruit and other citrus	Seed and segment	RP	½ inch	Pint jars: 10 Quart jars: 10
Peaches	Peel, halve, and pit	HP	½ inch	Pint jars: 20 Quart jars: 25
Pears	Peel and halve or slice	HP	½ inch	Pint jars: 20 Quart jars: 25
Pineapple	Peel and slice	HP	½ inch	Pint jars: 20 Quart jars: 25
Plums	Prick	HP or RP	½ inch	Pint jars: 20 Quart jars: 20
Rhubarb	Slice one inch thick	HP	½ inch	Pint jars: 10 Quart jars: 10
Tomatoes (packed in water)	Peel, pack whole or halves;	HP or RP	½ inch	Pint jars: 40 Quart jars: 45
Tomatoes (packed in juice)	Peel, pack whole or halves;	HP or RP	½ inch	Pint jars: 85 Quart jars: 85
Dill Pickles	Season according to recipe	RP	½ inch	Pint jars: 10 Quart jars: 15
Sweet Gherkin Pickles	Season according to recipe	HP	½ inch	Pint jars: 10 Quart jars: 15
Bread & Butter Pickles	Season according to recipe	HP	½ inch	Pint jars: 10 Quart jars: 15
Pickle relish	Follow recipe	HP	½ inch	Pint jars: 10 Quart jars: 15

◉ When the time is up, remove the jars and place them on racks, and follow the instructions above on cooling and labeling jars.

PRESSURE CANNING LOW-ACID VEGETABLES Pressure canning is a good method to preserve vegetables. Most need to be blanched first. Save the blanching water; it is rich with nutrients and can be used to pack the food in jars. Once the food is blanched, immediately pack in jars and fill with the blanching water, leaving a half-inch of headroom for all vegetables except corn, peas, and lima beans, which need one inch. You can also use boiling water. Follow the steps for prepping sealing jars carefully.

STORING CANNED FOODS The ideal temperature for storing canned foods is around 60°F. Store away from light. Keep an eye out for warning signs telling you that canned foods have spoiled. Do not eat or open any jar of canned food that leaks (or has leaked), foams, has a bad appearance, or has a metal top that has started bulging. Once you open a jar of canned food, if it smells bad or if you see signs of mold anywhere, discard it. If you must discard a jar of canned food, it is essential that you do so in a way such that no person or animal could possibly eat it. Never put it in the compost.

TRUE TIP

According to folk legend, leaves should be gathered when the moon is waning (the two weeks after the full moon), when leaves are said to hold the least moisture. Roots should be gathered when the moon is waxing (the two weeks before the full moon), when they are said to be at their most tender.

Drying Herbs

If you grow herbs, or can find them fresh locally, you can easily dry some for use in the winter. As with other foods, it is important to dry the herbs quickly to avoid losing flavor and nutritional value.

The flavorful oils in leafy herbs such as basil, marjoram, mint, and savory are the strongest just before the plant blossoms, so this is the best time to pick herbs for drying. Pick them early in the morning, which is when the leaves have the most oils. Using scissors, or pinching between your fingers, clip off the top of the plant. If the herbs need to be washed, rinse them quickly, spin, and then air dry.

The ideal temperature to dry herbs is 105°F. It is important to dry herbs away from sunlight, the darker the better. The most successful way to dry herbs is to hang them upside down, so that as much oil as possible migrates to the leaves. Hanging herbs upside down in a warm, dark, dry place, such as in an attic or upstairs closet, is ideal.

To hang herbs, wrap a string around the stems and tie in a knot, leaving at least 12 to 24 inches of string. Get a brown paper bag (this will keep the herbs from getting dusty), punch holes in it (make a lot of holes for adequate air circulation), and dangle the herbs in the bag, allowing the string to escape through the top of the bag. Use the string to tie the bag shut, with a bit remaining to tie to a rafter, nail, hook, or whatever is available.

If you use a food dehydrator or oven for herbs, try to regulate the temperature to around 105°F, and make sure there is air circulation.

Herbs are dry when the leaves crumble easily.

Can we believe food safety dates? According to the USDA, the dates stamped on the bottom of food packages are a good-faith promise of a food's safety until the specified time. There is no current uniform or universally accepted system of food dating in the United States, and the dates found on perishables are unregulated. (Infant formula and some other baby foods are regulated by the FDA, however.) Solution? Date your food yourself!

General Rules for Storing Dried Foods

Some people like to give dried food a "hit" of high heat, or a blast of freezing cold, at the very end of the drying

Cooking & Eating

DRYING YOUR OWN HERB SEEDS

For seeds that you collect for herbal use, like dill seeds or coriander seeds, here are the rules to follow: Pick the seed pods once they start turning brown. As with all herbs, pick them in the morning. Hang the stalks or pods to dry, as directed for herbs, inside brown paper bags. Once thoroughly dried, the seeds will fall and be caught by the bag.

process to discourage mold growth. To do this with heat, place the food on drying racks in the oven, at 175°F, for just 10 or 15 minutes. For the freezer, place the dried food in freezer bags or containers, and freeze for two or three days.

- Place dried food in airtight containers (glass jars with screw tops are ideal), and store it away from light, such as in a dark cabinet or closet. The best temperature for storage is a cool room temperature, around 60°F.
- Check the stored food every week or so, and give it a shake. If moisture condensation has developed, return the food to the drying process right away
- Dried foods can be frozen. Place in appropriate freezer containers. Freezing extends the life of dried herbs, for example, so you enjoy a flavor closer to fresh herbs for a longer time after the harvest.

Parsnip and Sweet Potato Fries

Getting tired of potatoes in the middle of winter? That's where parsnips and sweet potatoes come into play. Make oven-roasted "French fries" with these winter staples. The natural sugars in both transform in the magical alchemy of roasting to sweet and earthy, savory and subtle flavors.

1 pound parsnips
1 pound sweet potatoes (or 2 pounds of either one)
1½ tablespoons olive oil
Coarse salt and ground pepper

1. Preheat oven to 400°F.

2. For parsnips, trim tops and bottoms and peel. Slice in half crosswise so you have a thick piece and a thinner piece, then halve or quarter those until you have sticks of roughly the same size. For sweet potatoes, scrub and cut into sticks.

3. On two large baking sheets, spread out the parsnips and sweet potatoes in a single layer and toss with the olive oil, then season with coarse salt and ground pepper.

4. Roast until tender and caramelized on the edges, 25 to 40 minutes depending on thickness, giving the fries a stir about halfway through cooking.

REHYDRATING DRIED FOOD You can use dried food as is, or you can restore moisture to soften it and make it pliable. To rehydrate, place the dried fruit or vegetables in a bowl and cover with cold water. The longer they soak, the softer they get. Once the food is soft enough for your taste or use, remove it and use it as you would the equivalent fresh food.

Root Cellars

If you live in a climate where the temperature hovers around freezing or below in the winter, you may want to consider establishing a root cellar for yourself. In fact, if you live in an old house, you may already have one in your basement.

Root cellars are naturally cool and moist food storage areas, typically small rooms in the coldest part of a basement. Food keeps there because microorganism and enzyme activity are slowed or even halted at temperatures between 32°F and 40°F. The enclosed steps leading down into an unheated basement can be an ideal root cellar, for example.

A root cellar can keep bushels of fruit and vegetable crisp and fresh well into the winter. Some, such as sweet potatoes, can even be stored at a higher temperature, up to 60°F. Use a thermometer to find likely spots in your home or basement. You may decide to store some food in one place and other food in another, depending on temperature.

Without enough moisture in the root cellar, the food will get dehydrated, shriveled up, and ruined. For most foods, the humidity has to be really high, between 80 to 90 percent—virtually a rain forest! You can even place pans of water on the root cellar floor to raise the humidity.

To check to be sure your herb leaves, roots, or seeds have been fully dried, put them into an airtight jar and set them on a sunny windowsill for an afternoon. If moisture collects on the inside of the jar, they are not fully dry yet and might mold in storage. Put them back to dry some more.

I think of my root cellar as a secret underground garden into which I spirit away many of my crops when winter threatens.

—ELIOT COLEMAN, *THE NEW ORGANIC GROWER'S FOUR-SEASON HARVEST*

Long-lasting varieties of different fruits and vegetables are often called keepers—a distinction worth noting if you are stocking a root cellar. Ask local farmers which of their varieties keep the longest.

HOW TO STORE FOOD IN A ROOT CELLAR Harvest or purchase the produce when it is as ripe as possible, just before predicted first frost dates in the fall. Break off any leaves, such as carrot tops. Inspect carefully and only store undamaged produce.

Some vegetables should be cured—allowed to stand out in warm, open air to develop a tough outer skin—before they are placed in a root cellar. Onions, sweet potatoes, pumpkins, and winter squash should be cured on a sunny counter; potatoes and garlic in the shade.

Do not store different types of fruit or vegetables together in the same containers. Check root cellar produce frequently through the storage season, to remove anything that is going rotten.

Fun, Kids, Pleasure

BLACK ROCK FRUIT ROLL-UPS

Emily Zaas of Carroll County, Maryland's Black Rock Orchard makes roll-ups from fruit picked on her farm. First she makes an applesauce puree as a base, then adds other ripe fruit, such as summer raspberries. She pours the sauce onto mesh cloth and stacks the cloth on racks to dry. Her result: sheets of dried fruit.

Once the fruit mixture dries, she cuts the sheets into squares, lays them on sheets of plastic wrap, and rolls them up, sticking surprise quotes inside as if they were Chinese fortune cookies.

She sells these at green markets in the Washington, D.C., and Baltimore area, along with a wide variety of fresh fruit.

We should all seek food closer to home, in our foodshed, our own bioregion. This means enjoying seasonality and reacquainting ourselves with our home kitchens.

—JOEL SALATIN, POLYFACE FARMS, SWOOPE, VIRGINIA

Cooking & Eating

INGREDIENT SWAP

To maximize locally available ingredients, flex your recipes. A favorite recipe may call for raisins, but you live in apricot country—or you may be asked to use almonds, but you live down the road from a hazelnut farm. Don't be afraid to swap same-food-family items. Or get creative and substitute by taste and/or texture: For example, diced and brined roasted local peppers can stand in for capers, or soaked and salted raw sunflower seeds grown nearby can take the place of black olives grown in Europe.

Roasted Kale with Raisins and Pine Nuts

In Spain, spinach is commonly prepared with raisins and pine nuts. Try winter-friendly kale instead, oven-roasted, resulting in crispy leaves that melt in your mouth, with a subtle surprise of sweet fruit and nuts.

- 2 bunches kale
- 2 tablespoons oil
- ¼ cup raisins or any local diced dried fruit (apricots, plums, cranberries)
- ¼ cup pine nuts or any local nuts (almonds, hazelnuts, or try pumpkin seeds)
- Salt and pepper to taste

1. Preheat oven to 375°F.

2. Rinse kale and dry thoroughly. Remove and discard thick ribs and tear leaves into pieces, then dry again.

3. Spread kale on a large rimmed baking sheet and toss with oil and fruit.

4. Bake for 10 minutes, stirring every 5 minutes.

5. When leaves begin to crisp on edges, toss in nuts.

6. Cook another 5 minutes until kale is slightly browned and crisp, watching that nuts don't brown too much.

7. Season with salt and pepper.

SNAPSHOT **JOAN GUSSOW, ED.D.**

"I came to the conclusion that the only ecologically sound diet would be from foods available nearby, simply because of the transportation costs."

New York, New York

Professor emeritus, Columbia Teachers College

Author, *The Feeding Web; Chicken Little, Tomato Sauce, and Agriculture;* and *This Organic Life: Confessions of a Suburban Homesteader*

Joan Gussow was among the first to advocate eating locally and seasonally for environmental reasons. Like most visionaries, she was viewed as highly unconventional. Her ideas flew in the face of all the tenets of modern industrial agriculture, but they were based on enormous amounts of common sense and have since been enthusiastically supported by the sustainable farming community.

Gussow first advocated eating locally as a means of energy conservation. She observed that it takes a lot of gas and oil to transport food for thousands of miles, and it takes a lot more to keep it cold for all that distance. Locally produced food would not need to be refrigerated for such long periods of time, nor would it need to be shipped.

Gussow eats a diet of local and seasonal produce, and has found it to be relatively easy. She asks people to make a list of things they really don't want to give up and that can't be produced locally. She says that it is surprising how small a list it is. Coffee is always on the list. (She tells coffee lovers that coffee is okay for people to import as long as it is produced sustainably. Coffee does not weigh a lot and therefore takes less energy than many foods to transport, and it doesn't need to be refrigerated en route.) One person at a conference she attended added artichokes to the list, and a farmer announced that he was growing artichokes on his farm in Vermont! You'd be surprised what you can find locally.

Butternut Mac 'n' Cheese

Butternut squash might be one of the easier winter vegetables to get kids to love. Its bright hue and sweet flavor often please young palates, and this recipe is almost guaranteed to convert even the most veggie-phobic of children. It's a great one for parents, too, as most of the traditionally used dairy fat is replaced by the fragrant butternut puree.

- 1 small butternut squash (about 1 pound), peeled, seeded, and cubed
- 3 tablespoons olive oil, divided
- 1 pound whole wheat elbow macaroni (or your favorite pasta)
- 1½ cup vegetable stock
- 1 cup cheddar cheese, grated
- ½ cup part-skim ricotta cheese
- 4 tablespoons grated Parmesan cheese, divided
- Pinch of nutmeg
- Pinch of white or cayenne pepper
- ½ teaspoon coarse salt
- ¼ cup bread crumbs

These vegetables are traditional root cellar favorites: beets, carrots, celeriac, turnips, potatoes, sweet potatoes, winter squash, cabbage, garlic, onions, rutabagas, dried beans.

1. Preheat oven to 375°F.

2. Toss butternut cubes with 1 tablespoon olive oil and roast on a baking sheet until tender and edges start to brown, about 35 minutes.

3. While squash is cooking, boil pasta until al dente. Drain, sprinkle with olive oil, and return to pot off the heat.

4. When squash is done, mash it with a potato masher in a large bowl, adding vegetable stock until you have a thick, saucelike puree.

5. Stir pasta, cheddar, ricotta, and 2 tablespoons Parmesan cheese into the squash mixture. Season with nutmeg, pepper, and salt.

6. Lightly oil a deep baking dish (square 9-inch pan or equivalent). Add mixture.

7. Combine remaining Parmesan cheese with bread crumbs and 1 tablespoon olive oil and sprinkle on top.

8. Bake for 20 minutes covered with foil, then remove foil and bake for another 30 minutes or until browned and bubbling.

STEP 2

Eat a Variety of Foods

Include as wide a range of foods in your family menu as you can. By supporting diversity in food, you might help save a breed of animal from extinction, a seed with vital genetic diversity, or a plant that is resistant to rapid climate change. This important step will benefit your great-grandchildren—and, for the here and now, it will add a wide range of colors, flavors, textures, and nutrients to your diet.

WHAT IT MEANS

Choosing Food Diversity

The world provides a panorama of food possibilities. The more broadly you partake, the better.

Today just a few species of plants—primarily corn, wheat, rice, and tubers such as potatoes—provide 90 percent of the food grown, cooked, served, and eaten. Though there are hundreds—no, thousands and thousands!—of food products available in supermarkets, they are not made up of hundreds of different kinds of plants, but mostly just these few, rearranged in myriad different recipes and packages. As a result of the sameness—driven in large part by the industrial food production processes we have come to depend on—the variety of types within species is disappearing dramatically. For instance, in 1903 U.S. farmers planted and harvested 578 varieties of beans; some 80 years later, only 32 of those still existed, many of them protected in gene banks.

Learn more about the dangers of losing food plant diversity by reading *Shattering* by Cary Fowler and Pat Mooney. Learn more about efforts to save and share diverse food plants around the world by visiting the Global Crop Diversity Trust website: www.croptrust.org.

Unless we preserve diversity, our food supply is vulnerable. A monoculture of genetically uniform plants that lack disease resistance could result in a nightmare for the world, a catastrophe as devastating as nuclear war, some believe.

Such nightmares have already happened. The Irish potato famine, which killed thousands of people and caused millions to emigrate in the 1840s, was caused by the reliance on one kind of potato, which turned out to be vulnerable to a fungus that grew and spread during a particularly damp spell, wiping out all of Ireland's potato crops and contaminating the soil for decades. In the 1970s, such a nightmare threatened again. Southern corn leaf blight killed 15 percent, or a billion bushels, of corn in the United States, and U.S. seed exports may have spread the blight to Africa, Latin America, and Asia. The only way to avoid such global disasters is to support a variety of food grown with seeds rich in genetic diversity—and, better yet, to grow, save, and plant heirloom seeds here at home.

WHY IT MATTERS FOR YOU

The Value of Variety

For optimum health, we all need a broad range of nutrients from a variety of foods.

The wider the variety of foods in our diets, the greater the chance of getting all the nutrients we need, reports the FDA. Look upon Step 2 as your invitation to explore preparing and eating a wide range of roots, fruits, vegetables, leaves, stems, and seeds.

Nutritional variety comes from genetic diversity, too, and when you follow this step, you are also supporting the growing of true food, rich in genetic diversity. When farmers plant fewer varieties, consumers have less variety to choose from. That prospect has more dire consequences than simply fewer flavors on the supermarket shelf. Most agricultural plant breeding programs in the United States emphasize yield, uniformity, market acceptability, pest resistance, and transportability—not nutritional quality. In fact, breeding plants for the characteristics desirable for industrial production and marketing often lowers the plants' nutritional values.

Primal Seeds, a nonprofit diversity advocacy group, reports that according to the Food and Agriculture Organization of the United Nations, 75 percent of the genetic diversity of crop plants was lost during the 20th century. For example, Primal Seeds notes that Filipino farmers once grew thousands of kinds of rice. Today only two varieties account for 98 percent of the rice sown there. Mexico has lost an estimated 80 percent of its varieties of maize. And a survey conducted by the advocacy group Erosion, Technology, and Concentration (ETC) found that approximately 97 percent of the varieties ever listed by the U.S. Department of Agriculture had been lost in the last 80 years.

WHY IT MATTERS FOR EARTH

Agricultural Multiculture

Just as the fields and forests depend on the intricate interactions of many species, so do farms.

Martin Teitel points out in *Rain Forest in Your Kitchen* that farms in Chile have displaced their own native and traditional fruits and vegetables in favor of the same 15 to 30 species of crops grown around the world.

Research suggests that traditional agriculture depended on 80,000 species of plants worldwide. Industrial agriculture, with its ever broader reach around the world, now provides most of the food on our planet from just 15 to 30 cultivated plant species.

The importance of plant diversity shines through especially on an organic farm, without chemical and industrial technologies to mask the necessity for a balance of nature. To keep an organic farm in a thriving natural balance, the farmer must grow a diversity of plants, which helps keep the soil healthy. If the public will eat only a few commodities over and over again, there is no market for the organic farm's wider selection of produce.

The farmer's industrial counterpart, on the other hand, will be monocropping—growing a few commodities, sometimes just one—and while the market supports growing these few products, industrial farms can grow them only by using synthetic pesticides and fertilizers.

SAVING THE PLANET IN YOUR KITCHEN Making the choice to support a variety of local, seasonal food grown on local, sustainable farms has far-reaching implications. Great damage is done to the planet's genetic resources when we rely so heavily on so few plant varieties. When native crops are displaced by a small number of species grown for export, the survival of native peoples and their cultures are threatened with extinction as well.

The Importance of Seed Stewardship

Farmers and gardeners need not only to grow a wide variety of crops but also to choose with care the seeds they use. It has been said that a backyard gardener could save the world from famine. How? Every time you plant a garden, choose open-pollinated and heirloom seeds. Who knows which exact seed might be the one to withstand a global blight? If you think about it, that

Simple Stewardship

WE ARE WHAT WE EAT

Variety is one of the key principles at the heart of the slow food movement. "We believe that everyone has a fundamental right to pleasure and consequently the responsibility to protect the heritage of food, tradition and culture that make this pleasure possible," reads the statement of philosophy offered on the website of Slow Food, an international nonprofit organization. "Our movement is founded upon this concept of eco-gastronomy—a recognition of the strong connections between plate and planet." Everyone is not just a consumer but a "coproducer" of food, in that every choice at a restaurant, grocery, or farmers' market influences the world's agricultural production choices. Visit the website at *www.slowfood.com.*

same seed could just as easily have been lost because a family stopped growing and saving seeds of a plant variety, not knowing that they were the last holders of that seed on the planet!

The flavorful advantages of heirloom varieties will bring the importance of seed stewardship home to your dining table. Add an heirloom tomato to your salad—it may not look perfectly round, and it may not even look like other tomatoes plucked from the same plant. These are some of the reasons that industrial farmers don't grow heirloom fruits and vegetables: They are not bred to be grown in high densities, harvested mechanically, and marketed hither and yon, exactly predictable in shape, size, and color. All the more reason to save this esoteric tomato's seeds. Pass them on—by doing so, you may save one type of tomato from extinction.

A Tale of Three Seeds

Currently more than 300,000 seed samples are stored in the Svalbard Global Seed Vault in Norway—totaling more than 150 million seeds from global gene banks.

Many believe that the seed crisis is as urgent for the future of the planet as the threats of global warming and nuclear war. To understand it fully, we need to understand the differences among three kinds of seed: F1 hybrid, genetically modified, and open-pollinated heirloom. The first two types are sold by corporations, whereas heirloom seeds are passed down generation to generation. There are more than a thousand varieties of tomatoes that can be grown from heirloom seed, compared to the very few types of tomatoes produced from F1 hybrid. To illustrate the differences, let's follow three tomatoes: one from F1 hybrid seed, one from genetically modified seed, and one from open-pollinated heirloom seed.

SEED ONE—F1 HYBRID First-generation hybrids (also called F1 hybrids) are harvested from plants whose reproduction has been controlled by selective hand pollination. The seed stock is patented and owned by seed companies. These seeds are often sterile—you couldn't take a seed from a tomato or an ear of corn grown from F1 hybrid seed and plant it to grow more. These seeds are sold by multinational seed companies for the sake of an agricultural system that produces high yields of uniformly predictable produce. They have broad commercial appeal because the resulting produce is so uniform. When you sit down to eat a salad with a tomato that you bought at a supermarket, chances are that the tomato was grown from an F1 hybrid seed.

Like animals, plants result from the combination of male and female genetic material, but breeders make F1 hybrids by "selfing" plants—fertilizing a plant with its own pollen. The resulting seeds are genetically predictable, selected for traits suited to large-scale food production, yield per acre, uniformity of color and consistency, and pest resistance.

There are a number of problems hidden in the story of Fl hybrids. Many Fl hybrid seeds have unusual productivity for the first-generation plant, but after that their seeds become sterile or do not breed true, which means that farmers have to buy new seed every year, posing a serious financial challenge to many around the world.

Second, the tomato you buy today is most likely genetically identical to the tomato you will buy tomorrow, and the one you will buy next week. You will never get

Seed Savers Exchange is a nonprofit group dedicated to saving and sharing the heirloom seeds of our garden heritage. Their catalog is a sight to behold, full of a gorgeous array of plant possibilities that will enrapture your senses. Since 1975, Seed Savers Exchange members have passed on approximately one million rare garden seeds to other gardeners. Learn more at www.seedsavers.org. Or write Seed Savers, 3094 North Winn Rd., Decorah, IA 52101.

The loss of genetic diversity—silent, rapid, inexorable—is leading us to a rendezvous with extinction, to the doorstep of hunger on a scale we refuse to imagine.

—CARY FOWLER AND PAT MOONEY, *SHATTERING: FOOD, POLITICS, AND THE LOSS OF GENETIC DIVERSITY*

SNAPSHOT **AMY P. GOLDMAN**

"I can't count the number of times someone has tasted one of my melons for the first time and said, 'This brings back memories of my childhood.'"

Rhinebeck, New York

Advocate for heirloom fruits and vegetables
Author, *Melons for the Passionate Grower*, *The Compleat Squash*, and *The Heirloom Tomato*

Amy P. Goldman is a passionate gardener and seed saver. Her mission is to celebrate and catalog the magnificent diversity of open-pollinated varieties of fruits and vegetables, and to encourage conservation of old-time varieties. When she was writing her book on melons, she conducted a taste test of her favorite varieties at New York's Union Square Greenmarket. "There was almost a stampede," she says. "Until they tasted heirlooms, the crowd didn't know what they were missing." But the delight of melons that taste sublime is only one reason to grow heirloom fruits and vegetables. The other is that we need their germ plasm. It's their genes that will help us fend off the potato famines and corn blights of the future. Without their genetic diversity, we will be prey to ever more virulent pests and diseases.

the same variety of nutritional benefits from your tomatoes that you would get by eating different varieties.

Third, as more and more industrial farms around the world are growing F1 tomato plants, they are forcing out of the market the hundreds of diverse tomato varieties that have, over the course of centuries, adapted to drought, freezing, and blight.

Finally, when blights or fungi attack F1 hybrid plants, industrial farms often use huge amounts of pesticides. Yet pesticide- and fungicide-resistant strains of plant diseases are developing all the time, making this a vicious cycle that poisons, then diminishes, both our food supply and the environment.

SEED TWO—GENETICALLY MODIFIED Genetically modified organisms (GM, or GMO, crops) are created by inserting a gene from another plant or animal into a host organism and altering the offspring's genetic makeup to produce a desired trait. GMO plants have been designed for a wide variety of traits, from pest resistance to faster growth. The United States leads the way in genetic engineering, producing two-thirds of the world's GMO seed.

The Non-GMO Project, a nonprofit collaboration, quotes the following statistics: In 2007, GMO seeds accounted for 91 percent of soy, 87 percent of cotton, and 73 percent of corn grown in the U.S. Since 2008, virtually all of the U.S. sugar beet crop has been GMO; at least 75 percent of canola grown in the U.S. is GMO; and there are commercially produced GMO varieties of squash and Hawaiian papaya. All told, the Non-GMO Project estimates, GMOs are present in more than 80 percent of packaged products in the average grocery store in the United States or Canada.

To date, food scientists and farmers have focused GMO production on corn, soy, and canola. Engineered to survive massive doses of the ubiquitous herbicide Roundup, or to resist insects, these three GMO staples have now found their way into well more than half of all food on U.S. grocery shelves, from cake mixes to cornflakes. Soybeans and corn, including genetically modified varieties, are also making inroads in places like Mexico, Guatemala, and Brazil, threatening genetic diversity and contributing to already acute rates of deforestation by encouraging large, monoculture field agriculture of a type never attempted before.

Amy Goldman loves them all, but she is willing to name favorites. Two notable tomatoes: Big Rainbow and Sara's Galapagos. Two notable squashes: Queensland Blue and Winter Luxury Pie. Two notable melons: Petit Gris de Rennes and Fordhook Gem.

Many GMO critics worry about the future, pointing to the industry's inability to protect traditional crops from contamination by GMOs, which could mix in with the seed stock or pollinate nearby non-GMO fields. A 2004 Union of Concerned Scientists study found that at least 50 percent of traditional corn, 50 percent of soybean, and 83 percent of canola seed stocks in the U.S. were contaminated with GMO seed. British tests on vegetarian sausages and soybeans similarly found that 40 percent were contaminated with ingredients from GMOs.

Genetically modified soy and corn crops also threaten genetic and biological diversity. Though banned in Mexico, GMO corn seed has, alarmingly, made its way into the country's cornfields, threatening 9,000 years of maize cultivation that has created a vibrant, genetically diverse array of corn varieties. The U.S. has also introduced

Simple Stewardship

WHAT ISN'T GENETICALLY MODIFIED?

If you want to be sure you are not purchasing any food made with genetically modified ingredients, look for the "Non-GMO Project Verified" seal when you shop. The Non-GMO Project offers North America's only independent verification for products made according to best practices for GMO avoidance. The Project was created by retailers who wanted an easy, consistent way to help shoppers see which products were free of GMO ingredients. Don't confuse this seal with "GMO-free" and similar claims, which are not legally defensible; the Project's claim is bestowed only on products that comply with a comprehensive definition of non-GMO that considers every level of the food chain, all the way back to the seed.

Spaghetti with Cherry Tomatoes and Toasted Crumbs

This recipe from Amy Goldman has a cherry tomato salad at its heart. A one-hour waiting period after assembly of the salad allows the salt and vinegar to bring out the natural flavor of the tomatoes. SERVES 10

- 1 loaf rustic bread (for the toasted crumbs)
- ½ cup pure olive oil
- Salt and freshly ground black pepper to taste
- 4 cups (2 pounds) cherry and currant tomatoes, mixed
- 2 cups Sherry Shallot Vinaigrette (see recipe below)
- 1 gallon water
- ¼ cup salt
- 2 pounds spaghetti
- 3 green basil sprigs
- 3 purple basil sprigs
- ½ cup grated Parmesan cheese

1. To make the toasted crumbs: Preheat the oven to 350°F. Remove the crust from the loaf of bread and cut the bread into large dice. Pulse in a food processor until the pieces are small. In a large bowl, toss the bread crumbs with the olive oil, salt, and pepper. Spread the crumbs evenly on rimmed baking sheets and bake, turning frequently, until browned. Let cool while you continue with the salad.

2. To make the cherry tomato salad: Slice the cherry and currant tomatoes in half. Combine in a medium bowl with the Sherry Shallot Vinaigrette and let rest for 1 hour prior to serving.

3. Bring the water to a boil and add ¼ cup of salt. Cook the spaghetti until al dente, approximately 7 minutes, and then drain.

4. Cut the basil in chiffonade.

5. In a large bowl, toss the pasta with the cherry tomato salad.

6. Garnish with the Parmesan, basil, and toasted crumbs. Serve right away so the crumbs remain crispy.

Sherry Shallot Vinaigrette

- 2 finely chopped shallots
- ¼ cup sherry vinegar
- 2 tablespoons red wine vinegar
- 1 tablespoon balsamic vinegar
- Salt to taste
- 1 cup pure olive oil
- ½ cup extra-virgin olive oil

1. Soak the shallots in the vinegars and salt for 30 minutes.

2. Whisk in the oils. Taste and adjust.

genetically modified corn in Guatemala. In Brazil, the world's second largest soybean-growing country, where the crop is expanding fast, large farms are just as rapidly replacing biologically rich Amazon forest and savannah with soybean monocultures. Brazil had long been the source of GMO-free soy for Europe and other markets, but the country legalized genetically modified soybeans in late 2003, and its share of genetically modified soy is on the rise.

And what about that GMO tomato seed we were going to follow? According to the nonprofit group GMO Compass, no GMO tomatoes are currently being grown in the U.S. or Europe. A decade ago, the tomato was a symbol of GMO food because of the infamous GMO tomato called FlavrSavr, designed to lack a ripening enzyme and therefore have a longer shelf life. But the FlavrSavr has disappeared from the market, deemed a failure, and to date no GMO tomatoes have replaced it.

Learn more about the Non-GMO Project, which represents the belief that everyone deserves an informed choice about whether or not to consume genetically modified products. Visit their website: *www.nongmoproject.org.*

SEED THREE—OPEN-POLLINATED HEIRLOOM Heirloom plants are cultivars that have been passed down through generations. A cultivar is a variety of a plant developed from a natural species and maintained under cultivation. Many keep their traits through open pollination—that is, by the natural fertilization of nearby flowers by pollen, creating new seed—and others have been propagated through grafts and cuttings.

Open-pollinated seeds are constantly being modified in nature because the plants cross-pollinate with others in the locale. Called serendipitous crossing, it is the way that plants pass genes back and forth. The genes have been fine-tuned over centuries, responding to a variety of climate and soil conditions as well as adapting to blights

Simple Stewardship

HOW TO SAVE SEEDS

Adapted from Seed to Seed *by Suzanne Ashworth*

You too can preserve garden diversity. You begin with fruits and vegetables grown from heirloom seed. Seeds that are embedded in damp flesh, such as tomatoes, cucumbers, muskmelons, or ground cherries, require wet processing. Follow these steps:

- Remove the seeds. Large fruits are cut open and the seeds are scraped out. Small fruits are usually crushed or mashed. Some seeds need to go through a fermentation process that destroys microorganisms such as bacteria and yeast.
- Wash the seeds in a large bowl of water. Stir the mixture vigorously. Viable seeds tend to sink to the bottom; poor-quality seeds tend to float, so discard those. Pour the seeds through a strainer and wash under running water.
- Dry the seeds on a glass or ceramic dish, cookie sheet, window screen, or a piece of plywood.
- Don't dry seeds on paper, cloth, or nonrigid plastic, because they may stick. Spread them as thinly as possible. Stir them several times a day. Always remember that damage begins to occur whenever the temperature of the seeds rises above 95°F, so never dry seeds in the oven. Even the lowest settings can damage seeds.
- Never dry seeds in the direct sun if there is a chance that the temperature of the seeds will exceed 95°F. Always remember that the air temperature is often not the same as the temperature of the seeds. Even at air temperatures around 85°F, dark-colored seeds can sometimes become hot enough to sustain damage.
- Fans hasten the drying process; ceiling fans are ideal, and placing seeds on window screens is best of all, as they allow for excellent air circulation.
- Tuck your seeds in a dry, dark place in a paper envelope, clearly labeled. Enjoy the next season's harvest!

The Agricultural Biodiversity Weblog has developed a list of links to people and organizations that promote agrobiodiversity. Visit their website: *agro.biodiver.se.*

and pests, which makes the resulting plants capable of staving off a variety of threats.

Selection of favorable traits by generations of farmers and gardeners has led to the domestication of all our major food crops. Seeds survived in this way for millennia before chemical sprays and fertilizers existed. Modern farmers who caretake heirloom seeds almost always grow them organically. Whereas often an heirloom seed will be native to a region, heirlooms do not necessarily imply native species—immigrants carry their native seeds with them, both deliberately and by accident, and then those seeds become domesticated in new locales.

To do our part to protect biodiversity, we need to request local farmers and gardeners who sell at farmers' markets to offer us diverse foods. Knowing there is a market may make them more inclined to experiment. If you grow your own vegetables, choose open-pollinated and heirloom seeds, save the seeds yourself, and pass them on to others.

The genes passed on in heirloom seeds give life to our future. Unless the 100 million backyard gardeners and organic farmers keep these seeds alive, they will disappear altogether. This on-farm, in-garden kind of preservation is called in situ conservation, versus ex situ conservation, which takes place in gene banks. This is truly an instance where every backyard vegetable gardener can make a decision that will make all the difference in the world.

The era of the Wild Apple will soon be past: it is a fruit which will probably become extinct in New England.... He who walks over these fields a century hence will not know the pleasure of knocking off wild apples.

—HENRY DAVID THOREAU, "WILD APPLES," *WALDEN* (1862)

Roasted Heirloom Tomato Soup

Flavorful tomatoes spark up this traditional favorite, right through the end of their harvest—when the evenings grow cooler and the transition begins from salad season to soup season. SERVES 12

5 pounds mixed heirloom tomatoes, halved
2 bulbs garlic, ends sliced off but still in skin
4 medium leeks, washed well, dark green parts removed, the rest chopped into chunks
3 red or yellow peppers, halved and seeded
6 tablespoons olive oil, divided
6 cups water
1 cup red or white wine
2 cups tomato juice
3 tablespoons pureed sun-dried tomatoes
1 tablespoon paprika
1 cup basil leaves
4 cups milk (soy milk for vegan)
Salt and pepper

1. Preheat oven to 450°F. In a large bowl toss tomatoes, garlic, leeks, peppers, 3 tablespoons olive oil and salt to taste. Spread on a large baking sheet and roast for 45 minutes, until vegetables are soft and charred.

2. Let cool. Squeeze garlic out of skin and add, along with the roasted vegetables, to all remaining ingredients but the milk in a large pot. (Reserve a few basil leaves for garnish.) Bring to a boil, lower heat, and simmer for 30 minutes.

3. Add milk, then puree in a blender (hold cover on tightly), food processor, or immersion blender until completely smooth. Salt and pepper to taste, and garnish with reserved basil. May be reheated before serving.

Find more fascinating native American seed varieties through Native Seeds/SEARCH—the Southwest Endangered Aridland Resource Clearing House—on this website: *www.nativeseeds.org.*

HOW TO DO IT

Eat the Rainbow

This rule brings pleasure to the eyes, health to the body, and a better future to the planet.

You may have heard advice to eat the rainbow—try every day to eat fruits and vegetables of many different colors. The wider the range of colors you eat, the more antioxidants and phytonutrients (plant-derived nutrients), including flavonoids, vitamins, and minerals, you are including in your diet. Eating a variety of colorful fruits and vegetables improves your health and, according to the USDA, reduces your chances of cancer, heart disease, diabetes, hypertension, and other scourges of the modern industrialized diet.

Colorful Reasons Why

There is some solid nutritional science behind the idea of including something of every color group in your daily menu.

Consider this rule of thumb: Every day, eat 35 different kinds of food. Follow this principle, and you will be sure to eat the rainbow, and get plenty of variety and nutrition, too.

RED MEANS RICH IN LYCOPENE, an antioxidant proving to be a powerhouse against cancer. These foods include strawberries, tomatoes, apples, cherries, red grapes, raspberries, watermelons, red peppers.

ORANGE MEANS RICH IN BETA-CAROTENE, which converts to Vitamin A, good for the eyes. These foods include carrots, orange peppers, pumpkins, sweet potatoes, yams.

YELLOW MEANS RICH IN CAROTENOIDS AND LUTEIN, helpful for the eyes and in the prevention of cancer. These foods include cantaloupes, corn, summer squash, yellow beans, grapefruit, lemons, oranges, nectarines, papayas.

GREEN MEANS RICH IN LUTEIN AND ZEAXANTHIN, antioxidants helpful for the eyes, bones, and teeth, with anticancer properties. These foods include dark green vegetables, celery, honeydew melons, and kiwifruit.

BLUE AND PURPLE MEAN RICH IN THE FLAVONOIDS called anthocyanins and phenolics, good for the brain, memory, and cardiovascular health as a person ages. These foods include blueberries, red cabbage, concord grapes, eggplant, raisins.

WHITE MEANS RICH IN ALLICIN AND SELENIUM, both helpful for the heart and as a cancer preventative. These foods include bananas, brown pears, cauliflower, garlic, mushrooms, light-fleshed potatoes.

Shopping & Saving

FEDERAL AID FOR LOCAL VARIETY

The Farmers' Market Nutrition Program (FMNP) is part of the Women, Infants, and Children (WIC) program, which provides food, health care, and nutrition education to low-income pregnant women and their children up to five years old. Established by Congress in 1992, it provides fresh, local fruit and vegetables to WIC participants, encouraging them to use farmers' markets. If you know someone who may be eligible, let them know about it.

Commerce and conservation can and must be made compatible.... Global market forces, typically thought of as the cause of environmental problems, are now one of the great hopes for the living world.

—FROM THE MISSION STATEMENT, E. O. WILSON BIODIVERSITY FOUNDATION

Finding the Flavor of Variety

There are several ways to ensure that you and your family are eating a variety of foods. First of all, you can add new types of food to your menu. In place of meat at dinner, serve a protein-rich combination of grain and beans. Consider eggs for other meals besides breakfast. Look for breads and pastas made with grains other than wheat for a change. If you had cheese for lunch, prepare tofu for dinner. Explore new recipes and ingredients.

Another way of eating a variety of foods is to get to know heirloom varieties of grains, vegetables, and fruits. As examples of genetically diverse foods within these categories, with their kind permission we have excerpted some plant descriptions from two heirloom seed catalogs, Seed Savers Exchange and Bountiful Gardens.

Healthy for You

IS MY PYRAMID YOUR WAY OF EATING?

The United States Department of Agriculture (USDA) recently reconfigured the graphic representation of their dietary guidelines, and the new chart echoes the idea of eating the rainbow. MyPyramid of 2009, as it is called, is an indicator of what everyone should eat to gain and maintain optimum health. Whole grains, vegetables, fruits, fats, milk, and protein are recommended, and the chart represents the proportional amounts of each. Within each food type, there is a world of variety, so following this chart can mean branching out into flavorful, nutritionally diverse, and interesting foods.

See a full-color version of USDA's MyPyramid, along with variations for special needs such as for pregnancy, kids, and preschoolers, at *www.mypyramid.gov.* There is a menu planner tool and help on weight loss, too.

Simple Stewardship

GROW YOUR OWN GRAIN

Although not many backyard gardeners consider planting grain seed, the fact is that grains are among the easiest crops to grow. Planting and harvesting grains can be a new adventure for the home gardener. Many need little processing after harvest, and they bring beauty to the garden.

Go for Grains

Wheat, rye, oats, and brown rice are familiar and available, but a visit to the health food store or section of the supermarket will expand the list of grains with barley, buckwheat, quinoa, spelt, and millet. Search local farmers' markets and seed catalogs for new grains, too, including unfamiliar versions of the grains you already know and use.

RED LEAF GRAIN AMARANTH This is a beautiful grain variety with striking tan and red leaves and heads. Selected for leaf color over many years by Suzanne Ashworth, author of *Seed to Seed*.

JAPANESE MILLET Leafy with many grain-bearing tillers, millet offers excellent biomass, almost as much as corn, so some are looking at its energy potential. It will regrow after cutting, and it dries faster than Sudan grass. It is, however, difficult to thresh and clean for eating.

RED QUINOA Quinoa is a protein-rich seed used as a grain, but related to greens such as Swiss chard. This variety has unusually flavorful red seeds, with a nutty taste.

Wash quinoa carefully before cooking to remove saponin coating, which can be bitter. Rinse and drain five times or more. Quinoa has a short shelf life due to its oil content. Buy a small amount.

SNAPSHOTS **DAN BARBER**

"Sometimes giving in to nature can be the

Pocantico, New York

Chef and co-owner, Blue Hill and Blue Hill at Stone Barns

The farm at the Stone Barns Center for Food and Agriculture lost more than half its field tomatoes in three days in 2009, due to a late blight. Dan Barber wrote of the experience in the *New York Times*, excerpted with permission here.

According to plant pathologists, this killer round of blight began with a widespread infiltration of the disease in tomato starter plants. Large retailers like Home Depot, Kmart, Lowe's, and Wal-Mart bought starter plants from industrial breeding operations in the South and distributed them throughout the Northeast. (Fungal spores, which can travel up to 40 miles, may also have been dispersed in transit.) Once those infected starter plants arrived at the stores, they were purchased and planted, transferring their pathogens like tiny Trojan horses into backyard and community gardens.

In 2009 there were many more hosts than in the past, as more and more Americans have taken to gardening. Credit the recession or Michelle Obama or both, but there's been an increased awareness of the benefits of growing your own food. According to the National Gardening Association, 43 million households planned a backyard garden or put a stake in a share of a community garden in 2009, up from 36 million in 2008. That's quite a few home gardeners who—given the popularity of the humble tomato—probably planted a starter or two this summer.

What's the lesson here? If you're planning a garden (and not growing from seed—the preferable, if less convenient, choice), buy starter plants from a local grower or nursery. It is no better to plant a tomato plant that traveled 2,000 miles to your garden than to eat a tomato that traveled 2,000 miles to your plate. If late blight occurs in a small nursery, it's relatively easy to recognize and isolate.

Remember that when you start a garden, you become part of an agricultural network that binds you to other farmers and gardeners. The tomato plant on the windowsill, the backyard garden, and the industrial tomato farm are, to be a bit reductive about it, one very large farm. As we begin to grow more of our own food, we need to reacquaint ourselves with plant pathology

biggest victory of all.”

and understand that what we grow, and how we grow it, affects everyone else.

Government can help. The cooperative extension service is still active, but budget cuts have left it ill equipped to deal with a new generation of farmers. More extension agents in the field during those critical weeks in June might well have resulted in swifter, more effective protection of the plants: early detection of any disease requires a number of trained eyes.

The food community also has a role to play. To many advocates of sustainability, science, when it's applied to agriculture, is considered suspect, a violation of the slow food aesthetic. It's a nostalgia I'm guilty of promoting as a chef when I celebrate only heirloom tomatoes on my menus. These venerable tomato varieties are indeed important to preserve, and they're often more flavorful than conventional varieties. But in our feverish pursuit of what's old, we can marginalize the development of what could be new.... Breeders in regions vulnerable to late blight should be encouraged to select for characteristics that are resistant to it, in the same way that they select for, say, lower water demands in the Southwest. While they're at it, breeders could be selecting for flavor and not for uniformity, shipping size, and shelf life. The result will mean not just tastier tomatoes; it will translate into a food system with greater variety and better regional adaptation.

Healthy, natural systems abhor uniformity—just as a healthy society does. We need, then, to look to a system of food and agriculture that values and mimics natural diversity. The five-acre monoculture of tomato plants next door might be local, but it's really no different from the 200-acre one across the country: Both have sacrificed the ecological insurance that comes with biodiversity.

What does the resilient farm of the future look like? I saw it the other day. The farmer was growing 30 or so different crops, with several varieties of the same vegetable. Some were heirloom varieties, many weren't. He showed me where he had pulled out his late blight-infected tomato plants and replaced them with beans and an extra crop of Brussels sprouts for the fall. He won't make the same profit as he would have from the tomato harvest, but he wasn't complaining, either. Sometimes giving in to nature can be the biggest victory of all.

WINTER AKUSTI RYE A variety of rye from Finland, it produces nutritious grain and a large amount of biomass for compost.

TEFF The smallest food grain in the world, teff is a staple for much of Africa, especially Ethiopia, where it is used to make *injera*, a fermented, pancakelike bread. It's also used for hay and forage and in a fermented beerlike drink.

EARLY STONE AGE WHEAT Sometimes called einkorn, this grain is currently in limited production in the Bountiful Gardens research garden. A rare, high-protein wheat (18.3% in an Ecology Action test), it has two bearded seed rows to each seed head, with many seed heads per plant (up to 90 with wider spacings). It was originally a widely cultivated variety in Switzerland, Spain, and the eastern Caucasus, and reportedly cultivated 7,500 to 12,000 years ago. A venerable, quality food source much higher in carotene than modern wheats, though difficult to thresh and clean.

KAMUT WHEAT Also known as Polish Wheat or Astraakan Wheat. Very beautiful seed heads of silvery blue and kernels two to three times the size of modern wheats. Higher in protein, vitamins, and minerals than modern wheats. Some reports that it is less allergenic. Makes superior pasta and puffed wheat, but doesn't make bread. Probably originated in the Fertile Crescent.

To simplify the environment as we have done with agriculture is to destroy the complex interrelationships that hold the natural world together.

—CARY FOWLER AND PAT MOONEY, *SHATTERING: FOOD, POLITICS, AND THE LOSS OF GENETIC DIVERSITY*

Cooking & Eating

RENEWING FOOD TRADITIONS

Managed by Slow Food USA, Renewing America's Food Traditions (RAFT) is an alliance of food, farming, environmental, and culinary advocates who have joined together to identify, restore, and celebrate America's biologically and culturally diverse food traditions through conservation, education, promotion, and regional networking. The RAFT Alliance brings local farmers, chefs, fishers, agricultural historians, ranchers, nurserymen and conservation activists together to exchange information, tell the stories of regional foods and food producers, and create publications. Visit the Slow Food USA website to learn more: *www.slowfoodusa.org.*

Variety in Vegetables

The world of vegetables offers everything from spring spinach to summer zucchini to hearty fall pumpkins and winter squashes. The variety is there, but too many people are blithely ignorant of it—as anyone who has had to answer a grocery check-out clerk's question of "What's this?" will attest. Tomatoes, cucumbers, and iceberg lettuce are just the tip of the iceberg, so to speak. Vegetables come in many varieties with their own flavors and attributes.

BEANS: DRAGON'S TONGUE Dutch wax bean that has large six- to eight-inch cream-colored pods with thin purple stripes that disappear when blanched. Wide, crisp, and juicy stringless pods. Compact high-yielding plants.

BEETS: CHIOGGIA First introduced to American gardeners in the late 1840s from Italy. Uniquely beautiful flesh has alternating red and white concentric rings that resemble a bull's-eye. Very tender, nice for eating and pickling. Retains markings if baked whole and sliced just before serving. A spectacular variety.

CABBAGE: RED DRUMHEAD Fine, sweet flavor—probably the best of all red cabbages. Round to slightly flattish, deep purple heads, seven inches in diameter. Very hardy. Plant in early spring for autumn harvest. It can be an excellent winter keeper, surviving mild winters and coming to harvest in the spring. Widely adapted. Good in salads, when pickled.

Bountiful Gardens Seed Catalog is published by Ecology Action, a nonprofit organization committed to biointensive gardening methods. It offers a number of open-pollinated and heirloom seeds. You can obtain a copy of the catalog by writing to Ecology Action, 5798 Ridgewood Road, Willits, CA 95490 or by visiting www.bountifulgardens.org.

CARROT: DRAGON CARROT The finest, most refined purple carrot available. Sure to be a best-seller at specialty and farmers' markets. The reddish-purple exterior provides an amazing contrast with the yellowish-orange interior when peeled or sliced. Sweet, almost spicy flavor.

CHARD: RHUBARB CHARD Deep crimson stalks and leaf veins provide contrast to the dark green, heavily crumpled leaves. Unique flavor. Very ornamental.

CHARD: RAINBOW MIX CHARD Red, yellow, pink, purple, white—this is a mix of distinct chard varieties, resulting in a grand show, with unexpected color combinations when the seed is saved and replanted.

CUCUMBER: DOUBLE YIELD CUCUMBER Very productive pickling type developed by a home gardener and introduced in 1924 by Joseph Harris & Co. of Coldwater, New York, who praised it for "its wonderful productiveness," promising that "for every pickle that is cut off, two or three more are produced."

SPINACH: GIANT WINTER SPINACH A cold-hardy variety with large lance-shaped, slightly crinkled, medium-green leaves. Excellent for fall seeding for a crop in early spring; also can be planted in spring.

KALE: RUSSIAN RED Many consider this the hardiest and yet frilliest kale. Very beautiful purple and red oaktype leaves. Can survive weeks of heat in the garden.

LETTUCE: SEED SAVERS LETTUCE MIXTURE
A combination containing the following eight varieties: Amish Deer Tongue, Australian Yellowleaf, Bronze

---

Sweet Potato & Pecan Salad

If you don't have access to a wide array of heirloom potatoes, there are always sweet potatoes. This salad takes variety a step further with the addition of dried fruit and nuts—a great vegetarian side dish, but it can also partner with the salty, smoky flavors of barbecue. SERVES 12

- ¼ cup olive oil
- 2 tablespoons pure maple syrup
- 3 tablespoons fresh lime juice
- 2 teaspoons grated fresh ginger
- 1 teaspoon curry powder (more or less, depending on heat of your spice)
- 6 pounds sweet potatoes, scrubbed and cut into ¾-inch cubes
- 1 cup chopped green onions
- 1 cup chopped fresh cilantro
- 1 cup pecans, toasted and coarsely chopped
- 1 cup dried fruit (raisins, cherries, apricots, etc.)
- Salt and pepper

1. Whisk together olive oil, maple syrup, lime juice, ginger, and curry powder. Set aside.

2. In batches, or using an extra-large pot, boil or steam sweet potatoes for about 10 minutes, or until just tender.

3. Transfer sweet potatoes to a bowl and let cool to room temperature.

4. Add the remaining ingredients and gently toss with dressing. Let stand for a bit to allow the flavors to mingle. Season to taste with salt and pepper.

Simple Stewardship

GENETIC DIVERSITY & OUR FUTURE

Climate change represents the greatest single challenge agriculture has faced in its 12,000-year history. In an evolutionary blink of the eye in country after country, crops will face conditions never before experienced. In many regions, the coldest growing seasons of the future will be hotter than any before. It is predicted that in sub-Saharan Africa, the number of days of extreme heat will double. Soil moisture will drop. Growing seasons will effectively shorten. In some areas we'll need crop varieties with shorter maturities, and with greater heat and drought tolerance. We may need varieties that flower earlier in the day to protect vulnerable pollen from the midday heat.

The central question for humanity is how to get agriculture ready, because if crops don't adapt to climate change, neither will we. Given the fact that a new variety of rice, wheat, or corn might take ten years or more to breed, we really don't have any time to waste.

So what do we do? First and foremost, we protect genetic diversity, which will provide the natural means for crop adaptation to climate change. We collect the remaining diversity. We protect all crop diversity in good seed banks with a duplicate sample in the Svalbard Global Seed Vault. We secure this system financially, by establishing a sufficient endowment for each crop to guarantee conservation. We screen the collections for traits necessary for crop adaptation. We support responsible plant breeding—not just for the major crops, but for all important crops. And finally, we realize that we are all in this together. No country on Earth possesses the diversity it will need to adapt to climate change. Interdependence is the new biological reality. We will learn to cooperate, to conserve and share crop diversity globally, or we will learn what it's like to be hungry. Thankfully, we have positive options.

—Cary Fowler, Ph.D.
Executive director, Global Crop Diversity Trust
www.croptrust.org

Arrowhead, Forellenschuss, Lollo Rossa, Pablo, Red Velvet, and Reine des Glaces. A great way to try them all.

TOMATO: GERMAN PINK One of the two Bavarian varieties that originally inspired the Seed Savers Exchange, these tomato plants produce large one- to two-pound meaty fruits with few seeds and very little cracking or blossom scars. Full sweet flavor. Excellent for canning, freezing, and slicing.

Variety in Fruit

Fruit can include apples, pears, plums, oranges, grapefruit, melons, and strawberries, as well as dried fruit such as apple rings. With any fruit, there can be many varieties.

WATERMELON: BLACKTAIL MOUNTAIN Developed by Seed Savers Exchange member Glenn Drowns in northern Idaho, where summer nights average 43°F. Round nine-inch dark green fruits weigh 6 to 12 pounds. Sweet, juicy, crunchy, scarlet flesh.

MELON: BIDWELL CASABA MELON This melon hails from Chico, California. Grown by John Bidwell (1819–1900), a Civil War general and U.S. Senator who procured his seed from the USDA in 1869. An enormous melon, 12 to 14 inches long and 9 inches wide, weighing 12 to 16 pounds each. Sweet orange flesh. Very adaptable variety.

March 11. Sowed Cavolo Romano Paonazzo (purple cabbage) in lower divisions of the uppermost triangular bed. sowed Neapolitan cabbage in the division next above. & Cavolo Romano a broccolini (Cabbage) in the next above that. –THOMAS JEFFERSON, IN HIS GARDEN JOURNAL (1777)

MELON: COLLECTIVE FARM WOMAN An old Ukrainian variety first offered by Seed Savers Exchange in 1993. Smooth, round, seven- to ten-inch melons with yellowish-orange skin and extremely sweet and fragrant yellowish flesh. Ripens early in central Russia, and can even be grown in Moscow.

MELON: CHARANTAIS Considered by many to be the most divinely flavorful melon in the world. Smooth, round

SNAPSHOTS **CARY FOWLER**

"Like so many things in this world, the new depends on the old. Without the old varieties, the new varieties could not continue."

Rome, Italy

Executive director, Global Crop Diversity Trust

Co-author, *Shattering: Food, Politics, and the Loss of Genetic Diversity*

Cary Fowler oversees the Global Crop Diversity Trust, part of the Svalbard Global Seed Vault, the world's only global backup seed storage facility dedicated to preserving crop diversity.

Often called the doomsday vault, the Global Seed Vault operates much like a safe deposit box created to save seeds even amid nuclear or climate crisis. The vault is built undergound and located in Norway's isolated Svalbard Archipelago. The seeds are stored at -0.4°F (-18 ° C) and are expected to last for a millennium.

As Fowler points out, the new species "simply could not survive" without the old. "And herein lies the irony," he says. "In the long run, the future of agriculture and the very survival of crops depend not so much on the fancy hybrids we see in the fields, but on the wild species growing along the fence rows, and the primitive types tended by the world's peasant farmers in the centers of diversity."

melons mature to a creamy, grayish yellow with green stripes. Sweet, juicy, salmon flesh. Typically the size of a grapefruit, perfect for two people. Ripe melons have a heavenly fragrance.

The number of apple varieties available in the supermarket is growing, but there are still usually no more than six. What a tragedy this is! Visit *www.AllAbout Apples.com* for as many as 2,000 apple varieties! These lists include older antique apples, current popular apples, and newer varieties produced by some of the world's finest growers.

MELON: GREEN NUTMEG In 1863 Fearing Burr, Jr., described 12 melon varieties for the garden, and Nutmeg was ranked as one of "the very best." High yields of melons that weigh two to three pounds, very reliably, year after year. Wonderful aroma, sweet flavor described as having a unique spiciness.

Eggs

Today, most eggs available commercially are from a few highly specialized breeds of hen used by the poultry industry. On the other hand, more than half of the 70 breeds of chickens found in the United States are in danger of disappearing, according to a census conducted by the American Livestock Breeds Conservancy. Nineteen breeds are on the critical list. Of particular concern are five breeds developed in North America: Javas, Buckeyes, Chanteclers, Delawares, and Hollands. Look for eggs produced by heritage breed hens at specialty food stores, farm stands, and farmers' markets.

Variety in Protein

Look beyond meat and fish for protein. It can come from legumes and nuts, not just from animals. Try these less common beans, available from Seed Savers Exchange.

GOOD MOTHER STALLARD Introduced to Seed Savers Exchange members more than a decade ago by Glenn Drowns. Family heirloom that has been enjoyed for generations. Wonderful rich, meaty flavor.

Pumpkin Tamales with Cherry Mole Sauce

Fruit, vegetables, nuts, seeds, beans, chilies, cheese, spices, and even chocolate! All combine for a sublime meal. MAKES 24 TAMALES

24 corn husks (plus more for tying)

Pumpkin Tamale Filling

- ½ cup roasted pumpkin, pureed (or use canned)
- 2 teaspoons olive oil
- 2 leeks, washed and sliced, pale parts only
- 1 garlic clove
- 1½ cups cooked white beans
- ½ cup crumbled feta or goat cheese
- 1 pureed chipotle pepper in adobo sauce (or favorite hot sauce) to taste
- Salt to taste

Pumpkin Tamale Dough

- 2 cups masa harina
- 1⅓ cups warm vegetable stock
- 1 cup butter, softened
- 1 teaspoon salt (unless in masa)
- 1 teaspoon baking powder (unless in masa)
- 1 ½ cups roasted pumpkin, pureed (or use canned)
- 1 teaspoon cinnamon
- 2 tablespoons maple syrup

1. Carefully separate husks and soak in hot water for at least 1 hour.

2. To make the filling: If using fresh pumpkin, you will need a 4-pound pumpkin—try a sugar pumpkin or cheese pumpkin, less stringy than a carving pumpkin.

3. Preheat oven to 400°F. Remove seeds and strings, and peel and cut pumpkin into chunks. Bake until tender, then puree in food processor—if very wet, strain out excess water. Alternately, use canned pumpkin puree.

4. Heat 2 teaspoons olive oil in a pan over medium heat. Add leeks and garlic and cook until leeks are soft. Stir in beans, ½ cup pumpkin, cheese, chipotle, and salt to taste. Let cool.

5. To make the dough: Mix masa harina in a bowl with enough warm stock to make a soft dough—be careful not to make it sticky.

6. Beat butter in large bowl on medium speed until light and fluffy. Add masa harina and 1 ½ cups of

Monoculture is dangerous: monoculture of the mind, the kitchen, and the field.

—MARTIN TEITEL, *GENETICALLY ENGINEERED FOOD*

pumpkin mixture gradually. Blend until well mixed and light in color. Stir in cinnamon and maple syrup.

7. Use 24 large husks to wrap tamales and reserve smaller husks to tear into strips for tying the ends of tamales and for lining the steamer.

8. Pat husks dry and place on work area, with narrow end at bottom. Place about 2 tablespoons of dough in the center of husk and spread into 4-inch square. Leave room for folding.

9. Place a heaping tablespoon of filling down the center of the dough. Fold husk in half lengthwise, and wrap the other side around to enclose filling. Fold up bottom (the narrow end) of husk to cover the seam and tie a strip of husk around the tamale to hold it together. (The top can stay open.)

10. Add enough water to rice cooker or stockpot with steaming rack to simmer for 1 hour.

11. Line steaming rack with extra husks and stand tamales upright with open end on top, in rack. Use extra husks (or crumpled foil) to help tamales stand straight if there is extra room. Cover tamales with extra husks to help steam.

12. Cover and steam gently, about 1 hour. Let cool before serving. Serve with Cherry Mole Sauce.

Cherry Mole Sauce

- 4 dry ancho chilies, stemmed and seeded
- 4 cups warm water
- ½ cup light oil
- ½ cup roasted pumpkin seeds
- ½ cup almonds
- ½ cup dried cherries
- ¼ cup sesame seeds
- 4 whole canned plum tomatoes, drained
- 2¾ cups (or more) water
- 1½ ounces chopped dark chocolate
- Salt to taste

1. Cover chilies in a bowl with warm water and soak until soft, about two hours—reserve 1 cup soaking water and roughly chop chilies.

2. Heat oil in heavy skillet over medium-low heat. Add pumpkin seeds, almonds, dried cherries, and sesame seeds, and sauté until toasted, about 12 minutes.

3. Place mixture in food processor with chilies, reserved chili liquid, and plum tomatoes. Puree until almost smooth.

4. Return mixture to skillet and add 2 ¾ cups water. Bring to a boil while whisking. Turn heat down, add chocolate, and stir until melted.

5. Simmer until sauce darkens, about 15 minutes. You can add water, ¼ cup at a time, if sauce gets too thick. Salt to taste. The sauce can be made ahead and chilled; before serving, just stir over low heat until warm.

IRELAND CREEK ANNIE ENGLISH Heirloom grown since the 1930s on Ireland Creek Farm in British Columbia. Superb delicious flavor; makes its own thick sauce.

RUNNER CANNELLINI Larger than the traditional cannellini bean; preferred by chefs for outstanding, full-bodied, nutty flavor. Texture is potatolike, smooth and starchy.

VERMONT CRANBERRY New England variety, known before 1876. Sweet flavor. Great for salads and relishes.

PAINTED PONY A distinct variety of American origin. Excellent for soups; retains markings when cooked.

JACOB'S CATTLE Originally cultivated by the Passamaquoddy Indians in Maine, this is the standard for

Simple Stewardship

THE MANY WAYS TO SAY SQUASH

Most grocery stores offer only a few types of squashes—acorn, butternut, zucchini, for example. Compare that with the squash varieties listed in the Native Seeds/SEARCH seed catalog, all traditional crops in the region of the southwestern United States and northern Mexico.

Native Seeds lists 42 different squashes, from the large, long-necked Batopilas to the apricot-fleshed Mayo Blusher; from the flat, ribbed Peñasco Cheese to the multicolored Middle Rio Conchos. Each variety represents a particular squash, gourd, or pumpkin grown by Native North Americans for generations.

Seed stock for all these varieties is available from Native Seeds/SEARCH, a nonprofit organization working to preserve the traditional crops of the U.S. Southwest and northern Mexico. Visit their website at *www.nativeseeds.org*.

traditional baked beans in the northeastern United States. Also great for chili.

JACOB'S CATTLE GOLD Similar in all aspects to regular Jacob's Cattle except for the color. A stabilized cross between Jacob's Cattle and Paint.

For more on heirloom crops and heritage animals, visit the Sustainable Table website, *www.sustainabletable.org*. Sustainable Table celebrates local sustainable food, educates consumers on food-related issues, and works to build community through food.

Variety in Meats

Just as over-reliance on one type of potato can lead to catastrophe if it is susceptible to blight, so too are animal breeds vulnerable to dying out if a wide variety isn't maintained. Industrial farms have narrowed the number of animal stocks raised to a very few. Fortunately, a growing number of sustainable farmers are preserving agricultural variety and protecting biodiversity by raising "heritage" or "heirloom" animal breeds and crops, just as other farmers and gardeners are raising heirloom vegetables.

HERITAGE LIVESTOCK BREEDS Heritage breeds are to animals as heirloom varieties are to plants. They are traditional livestock breeds raised by farmers in the past, before the drastic reduction of breed variety that came with the rise of industrial agriculture. In the past 15 years, 190 breeds of farm animals have gone extinct worldwide; currently 1,500 others are at risk. In the past 5 years, 60 breeds of common livestock have gone extinct. In the U.S., a few main breeds dominate the livestock industry.

- 83 percent of dairy cows are Holsteins, and five main breeds comprise almost all of the dairy herds in the U.S.
- 60 percent of beef cattle are of the Angus, Hereford, or Simmental breeds.
- 75 percent of pigs in the U.S. come from only three main breeds.

- Over 60 percent of sheep come from only four breeds, and 40 percent are Suffolk-breed sheep.
- 99 percent of all turkeys raised in the U.S. are Broad-Breasted Whites, a turkey breed specially developed to have a meaty breast.

Heritage animals were bred over time to develop traits for adapting to local environmental conditions. Breeds used in industrial agriculture are bred to produce lots of milk or eggs, gain weight quickly, or yield particular types of meat within confined facilities. Heritage breeds are generally better adapted to withstand disease and survive in harsh environmental conditions, and their bodies can be better suited to living on pasture.

These livestock breeds represent an important genetic resource; when heritage breeds go extinct, their genes are lost forever. By raising heritage livestock breeds, sustainable farmers not only maintain variety within our livestock populations but also help to preserve valuable traits within the species so that future breeds can endure harsh conditions. There is no official definition or certification for "heritage" animals, but for a livestock breed to be truly heritage, it must have unique genetic traits and it must also be raised on a sustainable and/or organic farm. Heritage animals are well suited to sustainable farms since they survive without the temperature-controlled buildings and constant doses of antibiotics administered to the commercial breeds raised on factory farms.

TRUE TIP

A total of 117 different varieties of protein-rich heirloom beans are listed by the Seed & Plant Sanctuary of Canada, from Adventist, a type of dry bush bean, to Wolley Wonder, a type of pole bean. See lists at *www.seedsanctuary.com*.

Reducing the diversity of life, we narrow our options for the future and render our own survival more precious. It is life at the end of the limb. **—CARY FOWLER AND PAT MOONEY, *SHATTERING: FOOD, POLITICS, AND THE LOSS OF GENETIC DIVERSITY***

Does Variety Mean Exotic?

When you shop, don't confuse variety with the exotic. "Exotic" means from faraway places. If you live in Maine, fruit from the South Pacific will add variety to your diet—but the fruit had to travel 8,000 miles, a high cost in energy. And that tropical fruit, good for long-distance travel, has been favored at the expense of perhaps tastier, more nutritious local varieties. Instead, scour your own community for locally grown, seasonal varieties of food.

SNAPSHOT **MARTIN TEITEL, PH.D.**

"Diversity is a sound strategy for a healthy life in the kitchen, but also at the intersection of the culture outside of the home."

Boston, Massachusetts

Executive director, Cedar Tree Foundation

Author, *Genetically Engineered Food: Changing the Nature of Nature* and *Rain Forest in Your Kitchen*

Martin Teitel questions the idea that one must choose between changing personal lifestyle or engaging politically in the larger systems in order to change the world. "A bit of both is the best balance," he believes. "If you only recycle and have a green kitchen, a large number of issues are bypassed, such as how what you buy is marketed and packaged—serious issues that affect many people and the environment." A person can bypass neither politics nor the effort it takes to have "a safe, sane, and delicious kitchen." He points out that we can't continue to support two separate food supplies in the country, a healthy one and an unhealthy one, which has the power to destroy. "In regard to food, yes, I am my sister's keeper," says Teitel. "I can't just say, 'Yes, I am going to be healthy, but I'm not worried about you.'"

STEP

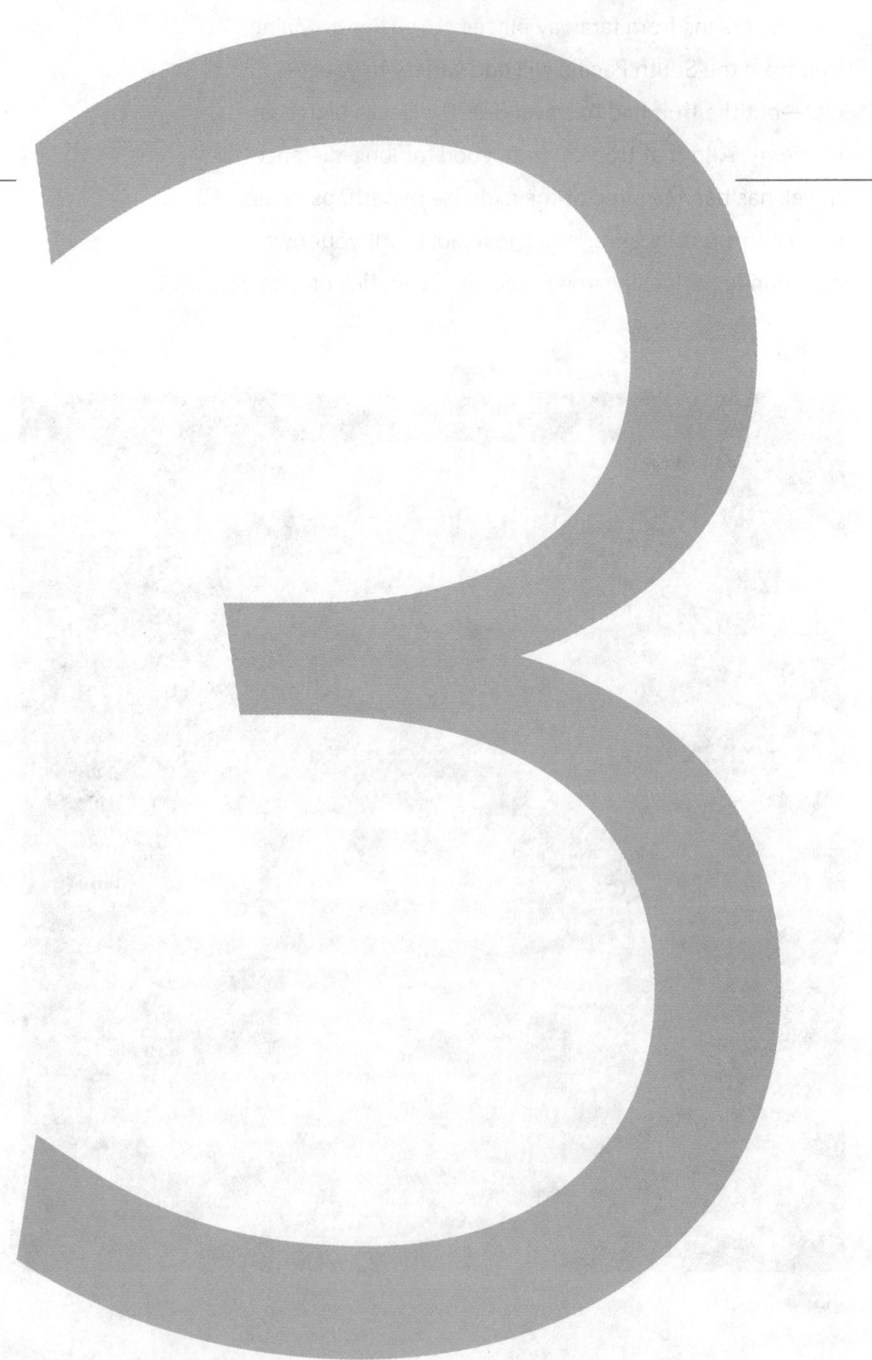

Aim for Organic

Purchasing and eating organic food confers far-reaching benefits—boosting not only personal health but also the health of farms, communities, and the environment. By supporting organic agriculture, we can limit the intake of synthetic chemicals in our bodies and in the environment and begin to restore the natural rhythms that come with growing and eating healthy food.

WHAT IT MEANS

Labels, Standards, Balance

Organic farming means both certified practices and cooperation with nature.

The word "organic" on a label identifies a product that comes from a farm where organic methods are practiced. In 2002 the U.S. Department of Agriculture (USDA) issued the first national organic standards and provided a product seal identifying and verifying food grown on "certified organic" farms. The standards set out the methods, practices, and substances used in producing and handling crops, livestock, and processed agricultural products. The standards include a national list of approved synthetic substances; the standards also prohibit a few natural pesticides that are highly toxic. But labels and standards tell only part of the story. Organic farmers would probably distinguish conventional farming from organic farming another way: Organic farming is about cooperating with nature rather than controlling nature. Productivity is achieved through nutrient recycling, which nourishes the soil, instead of with synthetic nutrients (fertilizers), which spike the soil.

Organic farmers seek to maintain and enhance ecological balance. The aim of an organic farm is to align itself with the land's natural ecology rather than to divide nature into camps of good and bad species. Indeed, the word organic suggests the integration of parts into a healthy, balanced whole.

Long before science could tell us why certain farming methods would produce greater crop yields, organic farmers were learning what worked and what didn't.

—DAVID SUZUKI, *THE NATURE OF THINGS*

WHY IT MATTERS FOR YOU

Perspective on Pesticides

Unfortunately, pesticides don't always end up on pests—they can land on the food you'll soon eat.

Organic fruits and vegetables contain only about a third as much pesticide residue as conventionally grown food, according to Brian Baker and Ned Groth, senior scientists at Consumers Union. Why does organic food contain *any* such residue? From past soil contamination or drift from conventional farms. Where there is pesticide spray, there is drift: Less than 0.1 percent of pesticide applied to crops reaches the target pest. The rest goes into the air, rivers, and living organisms.

But does it matter? According to a National Academy of Sciences (NAS) report, the answer is a resounding yes. More than 80 percent of commonly used pesticides today have been classified by NAS researchers as potentially carcinogenic. Indeed, some attribute increased rates of birth defects and human reproductive problems to the heavy reliance on pesticides by conventional farmers.

Infants and children are most vulnerable, which is especially worrisome given that in the U.S. some 20 million youngsters age five and under consume an average of eight pesticides daily. While Congress has tightened standards for residue levels allowed in common fruits and vegetables, an organic product carries fewer pesticides.

Among wildlife, there is also evidence that pesticides can mimic and block the action of naturally occurring hormones. Fish, frogs, and other aquatic animals eat or absorb persistent pesticides in waterways, which can affect them and the organisms that feed on them. Some pesticides concentrate in the tissues of organisms, causing the biggest problems in animals at the top of the food chain, such as birds, fish, and people.

According to the Environmental Working Group, some fruits and vegetables routinely carry less pesticide: onions, avocados, pineapples, mangoes, kiwifruit, asparagus, bananas, cabbage, broccoli, and eggplant.

WHY IT MATTERS FOR EARTH

An Ecological Balance

Sustainable agriculture replenishes the soil and recycles resources.

According to a 21-year Swiss study published in the May 31, 2002, issue of *Science Daily*, organic farming increases soil fertility and diversity of species. Organic agriculture also requires less water per hectare than do conventional farms and emits 40 to 60 percent less global-warming carbon dioxide, the Soil Association of Britain reported in 2000. Studies show that organic farming uses 70 percent less energy than industrial farming. "This energy conservation is achieved by recycling nutrients to maintain fertility, and using natural ecological balances to solve pest problems," says North Dakota organic farmer Fred Kirschenmann.

Environmental pollution and degradation, such as tainted drinking water, soil erosion, and loss of natural resources, are also linked to the use of toxic and persistent chemicals in farming. The U.S. is facing the worst topsoil erosion in history due to current agricultural practices of chemical-intensive, monocrop farming. The Natural Resource Conservation Service estimates more than 3 billion tons of topsoil disappear from U.S. croplands each year—25 billion tons globally. "We've lost well over half of our topsoil, and most of that has been just in the last 17 years," laments Kirschenmann. However, he observes, "damage to farmland from conventional farming is reversible by implementing sustainable farming practices."

Farms selling certified organic food are inspected annually and must provide a written plan of their organic management techniques. Farmers supply detailed records of diversity, practices for replenishing the soil, recycling of farm materials and resources, and humane treatment

Theo Colborn, Dianne Dumanoski, and John Peter Meyers report in Our Stolen Future that wild creatures around the world are experiencing disruptions in normal hormonal patterns and immune responses. Pesticides are high on the list of suspects thought to be responsible.

of farm animals. In order to be certified, agricultural products must have been grown on land that has gone through a three-year transition period when no substances prohibited for organic certification have been used. Records must also be kept for those three years.

HOW TO DO IT

Look for the Label

There are a lot of choices and options when you're buying organic food.

The standards issued by the USDA in 2002 gave consumers for the first time a "third-party verified" seal of certified organic food. This action

Fun, Kids, Pleasure

REPELLING LARGER CRITTERS

Sometimes it's the larger pests that wreak havoc in your garden. Here are some tips for keeping them away from your plants.

- Hang aluminum pie pans from trees. They shake with the wind, startling animals.
- Hang soap bars from trees or strew on the ground to ward off deer.
- Wrap dog or human hair in cheesecloth and hang near the garden.
- Build wire cages around bulbs to protect them from deer and mice.
- Moles don't like castor oil, so place bowls filled with ½ cup castor oil and 2 cups water around lawn and garden, or grow castor bean plants.
- Grow mint if you have a problem with mice.
- Make a spicy hot pepper infusion spray to deter squirrels.

followed 12 years of public discussion, after the U.S. Congress adopted the Organic Foods Production Act in 1990. The USDA's action offers consumers the assurance that all food products labeled as organic in the United States are governed by consistent standards. The organic standards implemented in 2002 allow different labeling options based on the percentage of organic ingredients in a product. These include three distinct categories:

100 PERCENT ORGANIC Only products that have been produced using exclusively organic methods and contain only organic ingredients (excluding water and salt) are allowed to carry a "100 percent organic" label.

ORGANIC To be labeled "organic," a product must contain at least 95 percent organic ingredients by weight, excluding water and salt, and the rest can only be natural or synthetic ingredients unavailable in organic form. The product cannot combine organic and nonorganic ingredients. For instance, if a loaf of bread is made with organic wheat, all of the wheat in the bread must be organic.

Healthy for You

HANDS-ON PEST CONTROL

- Pick bugs off the plant.
- Place paper collars around plant stems.
- Wrap tree trunks in heavy paper or poster board and brush with a sticky substances such as honey to trap bugs.
- Scatter broken eggshells. They are a deterrent to many slugs.
- Vacuum bugs off houseplants with a vacuum cleaner.
- Use soap spray, a favored folk pesticide. It disrupts cell membranes and dehydrates insects. See recipes on pages 98-99.

MADE WITH ORGANIC Products with 70 to 95 percent organic ingredients may display "Made with organic [up to three specific organic ingredients or food groups]" on the front panel.

A fourth category includes products that contain less than 70 percent organic ingredients. These can be labeled with an ingredient list that identifies those items clearly as organic, but the main panel of the product's label cannot say "organic."

The National Organic Standards Board, part of the Organic Trade Association, maintains a National List of Allowed and Prohibited Substances. For more on this North America-based trade association, see its website at *www.ota.org.*

Cost of Certified Organic Food

There is no way around it—certified organic produce and animal products cost more than nonorganic products. There is one big exception to this rule, however, and that is certified organic *packaged* food. In fact, organic meals, not including fresh produce, are actually comparably priced to meals prepared with conventional products. Some organic food—cheese, for example—does indeed cost more than its conventional counterpart, but the organic crackers you might put the cheese on are significantly cheaper than conventional crackers. The prices average out over a day's meals.

There is more to the economics of buying organic than the sticker price, however. There are many hidden environmental costs of industrialized farming. Choosing organic food means not passing the cost along to future generations, as happens with food from many other farms. You might say that paying more for organic food means investing—buying futures—in the environment.

Sustainable farms pay the full cost in this generation now, whereas factory farms charge some of their expense to the next generation.

—DAVID PODOLL, ORGANIC TURKEY FARMER, PRAIRIE ROAD ORGANIC FARM, FULLERTON, NORTH DAKOTA

Natural Pest Repellents

All-Purpose Insecticidal Soap Spray

Castile soap is used here as a totally organic method of removing insects from fruits and vegetables. It kills pests by dehydrating them.

1-2 tablespoons liquid castile soap
1 gallon water

Combine ingredients in a pan. Transfer 2 cups to a spray bottle. Spray infested areas. Do not use more than 2 tablespoons of soap; too much can kill the leaves.

Note: Detergent soaps will harm your plants. Use liquid vegetable-oil castile soap, sold at health food stores and many drugstores.

Garlic Spray

You already have an organic pesticide in your kitchen—garlic! Garlic has amazing pest repellent qualities, keeping many different kinds of insects at bay, as well as other pests that can destroy your favorite plants.

1 garlic head
2 cups boiling water
2 cups room-temperature water

Peel and mash the garlic. Place it in a pint mason jar and cover with boiling water. Screw on the lid and let set overnight. Strain. Freeze 1 cup of the infusion to use another time; put the rest in a spray bottle with 1 more cup of water. Spray on infested areas.

VARIATIONS

SOAPY: Add 2 teaspoons vegetable oil and 1 teaspoon liquid castile soap to the garlic infusion before dividing the batch in two.

SPICY: Combine any of the following in the garlic infusion: scallions and onions, horseradish root, ginger, rhubarb leaves, cayenne and other peppers. Add 1 teaspoon liquid castile soap.

ONIONY: Combine an onion and a few hot peppers with the head of garlic in a blender with enough water to cover. Strain. Freeze what you don't use.

Washing Soda

Here is another homemade pest repellent for your herbs, fruits, and vegetables, as well as for your favorite houseplants and flowers. Most pests don't like washing soda—a caustic, alkaline mineral.

1 teaspoon washing soda
1 teaspoon liquid castile soap
1 gallon water

Combine ingredients in a pail and stir. Pour some on infested areas, or put a few cups at a time in a spray bottle. Keep this in a covered container; its shelf life is indefinite.

Dormant Oil and Soap Spray

This is a popular spray in organic orchards, used in winter and spring. The oil suffocates insects. Most versions of dormant oil spray are made with a heavy petroleum oil, a nonrenewable resource, so we suggest you substitute vegetable oil.

½ cup vegetable oil
1 tablespoon liquid castile soap
2 quarts water

Combine ingredients in a pail. Transfer 2 cups to a spray bottle. Spray infected areas.

Banana Traps

Next time you eat a banana, save the peels to make a useful trap for some of the pests roaming your garden, especially slugs.

1 cup vinegar
1 cup sugar
A few chopped banana peels
1 gallon water

Combine ingredients and leave in open bowls or jars around the garden. Insects and slugs attracted to the smell will drown.

VARIATIONS

MOLASSES: Instead, combine ½ cup blackstrap molasses, 1 package active dry yeast, and 1 gallon water with chopped banana peels.

BEER: Substitute beer for water.

Many smaller farms do not go through the procedure of organic certification, yet they are growing food organically. Get to know the growers in your area by asking about their farming methods, how they raise their animals, and when and why they use pesticides.

Certified Organic Produce

Organic and conventional produce often look different. Organic produce may vary in size, be less uniform in shape or color, or be mottled or blemished. Chemicals in conventional agriculture are used not only to fight pests but also for cosmetic purposes—to enhance color, firmness, roundness. Some 10 to 20 percent of insecticides and fungicides are applied simply to comply with cosmetic standards. Organic produce is more perishable—and picked closer to ripeness. For example, lettuce, tomatoes, and beans should be eaten within days of purchase.

Meat, Eggs, and Dairy Products

For meat, eggs, and dairy, certified organic is the best choice. To be considered organic by a certifying organization, animals must be fed 100-percent certified-organic feed, forage, and hay. This eliminates the risk of mad cow disease (bovine spongiform encephalopathy), acquired from animal-based feeds. It also means fewer pesticides in milk or meat, since none are allowed in growing feed. If you can't buy organic, here are some questions to ask:

Simple Stewardship

SEAL OF APPROVAL

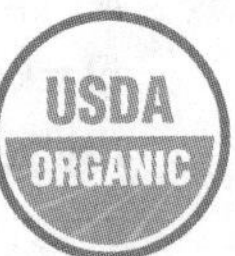

To assist consumers, USDA has designed a seal that may be used only on products labeled as “100 percent organic” or “organic.” Use of the seal is voluntary. Grocery stores are increasingly using the seal in their own shelf signage along with other point-of-purchase materials to help identify organic products. Nonfood products that meet the requirements for using the seal can also display it.

SNAPSHOT **FRED KIRSCHENMANN**

"What better way to ensure a healthy environment than to support organic farms that care for soil and water?"

Medina, North Dakota

Organic farmer

Distinguished Fellow, Leopold Center for Sustainable Agriculture

Fred Kirschenmann is one of sustainable agriculture's most eloquent spokespeople. He received a Ph.D. in philosophy from the University of Chicago, but his devotion to sustainable farming practices compelled him to become a full-time farmer. On his family's 3,500-acre farm in North Dakota, he pioneered organic farming techniques. He also founded Farm Verified Organic, Inc., a private certification agency, as well as the Northern Plains Sustainable Agriculture Society. He has also served on the USDA's National Organic Standards Board. Organic farms should be recognized for their positive impact on the environment, soil quality, and the ecology of neighborhoods, says Kirschenmann. "It is important to understand that what we are involved in here is a fundamentally different way of producing food, which has important social and political consequences for us all." Far more than just providing safe food, organic food supports an ecologically sound way of eating.

⊙ WAS THE ANIMAL FED ONLY GRASS AND/OR 100-PERCENT VEGETARIAN GRAIN?

A USDA labeling program for grassfed animal products is not helpful. Instead, look for the Food Alliance Certified or the American Grassfed Association mark, indicating the farmer adheres to clear standards. In both, the animals have spent most of their lives on pasture. For grassfed nonruminants, including pigs and poultry, grass is a major part but not the whole of their diet, since they also consume grains. The term "free range" is not a reliable claim.

For help in cutting costs, try Menu Planning Central or the Healthy Menu Mailer at *www.naturemoms.com/blog/about-tiffany.*

Grassfed animal products have been shown to be higher in beta-carotene (Vitamin A), conjugated linoleic acid (CLA), and omega-3 fatty acids, good for reducing cholesterol, diabetes, cancer, high blood pressure, and other life-threatening diseases. These products are lower in fat, cholesterol, and calories, and risk of infection by *E. coli* bacteria is virtually eliminated.

Late Summer Chili

This recipe relies on the bumper crop of late summer produce, and it is a chili—but a bright one light enough to handle the season and made with a colorful palette. **SERVES** 8

- 1 tablespoon olive oil
- 2 shallots, peeled and diced
- 3 cups red, yellow, or orange tomatoes, roughly chopped
- 2 carrots, scrubbed, trimmed, and sliced
- 1 ear of corn, shucked
- 1 large beet, scrubbed, ends removed, and cubed
- 1 large sweet potato, scrubbed and cubed
- 2 red, yellow, or orange bell peppers, seeds and ribs removed, diced
- 1 red chile pepper, seeds removed, and diced
- 1 cup canned organic cannellini (or other white) beans and liquid
- 1 teaspoon ground cumin (or to taste)
- Sea salt, to taste
- Fresh cilantro

1. In a large pot, sauté shallots in olive oil over medium heat until tender.

2. Add tomatoes and sauté until they start to release some of their juice.

3. Add in the rest of the vegetables and beans and bring to a simmer, stirring occasionally.

4. Turn heat down and let simmer until thick, about an hour. Depending on the mix of your ingredients, you may need to add a little water during cooking for the right consistency.

5. Stir in cumin and salt.

6. Serve in bowls and garnish with chopped cilantro.

Healthy for You

TOP TWELVE TO BUY ORGANIC

The following fruits and vegetables were found to be the most often contaminated by pesticide residues. Since it's not possible to eat organic produce 100 percent of the time, this list might help you prioritize for buying organic. The produce more likely to be contaminated is listed first.

- peaches
- apples
- bell peppers
- celery
- nectarines
- strawberries
- cherries
- kale
- lettuce
- imported grapes
- carrots
- pears

Source: The Environmental Working Group

⊙ WERE GROWTH HORMONES USED?

Two-thirds of the beef cattle raised in the U.S. are implanted with growth hormones. Although meat products contain only trace amounts of hormones, agricultural runoff of both hormones and antibiotics threatens the reproductive capabilities of fish in U.S. waterways.

If you can't buy organic meat products, look for those bearing one of these other labels: Certified Humane Raised and Handled, Food Alliance Certified, Animal Welfare Approved, American Grassfed Association. These programs do not allow growth hormones to be used.

For dairy products, if you can't buy certified organic milk, yogurt, or cheese, buy those with "rBGH-Free" on the label. Recombinant Bovine Growth Hormone (rBGH) is injected into cows to make them produce 10 to 20 percent more milk. The hormone elevates levels of insulin-like growth factor-1 (IGF-1), which can cause cell division and tumor growth, and may lead to breast and prostate cancer.

To find grassfed meat producers near you, consult the list of producers compiled by the American Grassfed Association website at *www.americangrassfed.org/aga-producer-members.*

SNAPSHOT **MERYL STREEP**

"As a new mom, I became aware of the importance of organic."

New York, New York

Oscar-winning actress

Cofounder, Mothers & Others for a Livable Planet

Meryl Streep's children were very young in 1989, when she and Wendy Gordon started Mothers & Others. They were responding to a report published by the Natural Resources Defense Council showing young children were being exposed to levels of pesticides in common fruits and vegetables that exceeded government safety levels. "I wanted what every parent wanted—to know what was the safest, best food to feed my children," says Streep. Organic food was not then widely available, and it was often more expensive. "My strategy then—and I think it still makes sense today—was to seek out and buy the organic version of food my kids loved, like apple juice and bananas and milk and chicken. I bought less processed foods, which ounce for ounce I found to be more expensive and less healthy than making it myself from scratch, and in season I bought fresh produce from the farmers' market in my town. My food budget never really changed, but what I spent it on definitely improved. And I knew that my kids were eating food that was safer for them, produced without pesticides, growth hormones, and antibiotics."

⊙ WERE ANTIBIOTICS ROUTINELY GIVEN?

Conventional cattle receive heavy doses of antibiotics in food and as treatment when they get sick. Animals raised on industrial farms receive on average up to 30 times more antibiotics than people do, some to treat or prevent infections but others to make them grow faster. Such overuse of antibiotics has contributed to a rise in drug-resistant bacteria in humans. Much more virulent strains of bacteria, such as *E. coli* O157:H7, have developed resistance to antibiotics.

If you can't buy organic meat, look for these other labels: Certified Humane Raised and Handled, Food Alliance Certified, Animal Welfare Approved, American Grassfed Association. These programs only allow antibiotics to be given to sick animals.

◉ WERE THE ANIMALS CONFINED?

If organic is not available or too expensive, but you want meat that comes from animals that spend their lives on pasture, look for products bearing one of the labels mentioned above: Food Alliance Certified, Animal Welfare Approved, American Grassfed Association.

Don't be misled by the term "free range." The USDA defines free range only for chickens, not eggs or beef, and access to the outdoors, according to their definition, can be as little as five minutes per day.

With the boom in organic foods, organic store brands are available in most supermarkets, bringing the cost of organic products down as much as 25 percent.

Cooking & Eating

MAKE YOUR OWN BABY FOOD

Equipment

Large pot or saucepan
Steaming insert (such as colander)
Baking dish
Blender
Ice tray (optional)

1. Cook your family's favorite fruit or vegetables until soft. Steaming maintains the most nutrients. Steaming, baking, and boiling all allow for big batches to be made.

2. Place the cooked produce into the blender, saving the liquid that they were cooked in. (For babies under seven months, do not use water from these high-nitrate veggies: carrots, spinach, beets, cabbage, broccoli. Substitute formula, breast milk, or plain water.)

4. Set your machine to puree or grind to mash the produce.

5. Gradually add liquid to make a puree of the desired consistency.

6. If desired, pour cooled puree into ice tray and freeze in portions.

Source: *www.wholesomebabyfood.com*

Reading the Labels

IF THE LABEL SAYS	IT MEANS	3RD PARTY VERIFIED
Demeter Certified Biodynamic *demeter-usa.org*	no synthetic pesticides, pastured livestock, well-managed agriculture	x
USDA Organic *ams.usda.gov/nop*	no hormones, antibiotics, genetic engineering, radiation, synthetic pesticides, or fertilizers	x
Fair Trade Federation Measures *fairtradefederation.org*	commitment to biodiversity-enhancing agriculture, humane labor practices, and other fair trade	
Fair Trade Certified *transfairusa.org*	assurance that farmers received fair prices for crops used in product	
Non-GMO Project Verified *nongmoproject.org*	ingredients do not contain more than 0.9% genetically modified organisms	
Treated with Irradiation	exposed to ionizing radiation to reduce pathogens	x
Rainforest Alliance Certified *rainforestalliance.org*	grown by farmers following sustainable practices to protect rain forest cover	x
Low-Input Viticulture and Enology (LIVE) *liveinc.org*	wine only; natural pest management, replacing chemicals with beneficial flora and fauna	x
Bird Friendly *nationalzoo.si.edu/ConservationAndScience/MigratoryBirds/Coffee/*	coffee only; grown by farmers committed to protecting tropical bird habitats	x
Grown Locally labels *localharvest.org*	meat and produce raised within approximately 100 miles of store	
Country of Origin labels *ams.usda.gov*	indicates country where product was raised	

Strawberry and Hazelnut Salad

Strawberries always star in spring and summer desserts, but they can be entirely effective in savory dishes as well. Once strawberry season has passed, try this recipe with other fruits. (Pears are heavenly.) SERVES 2-4

- 1 pint fresh organic strawberries
- ⅓ cup hazelnuts, lightly toasted and roughly chopped
- Shaved aged cheese

Rinse and hull berries, place in a bowl, top with hazelnuts, garnish with cheese. Drizzle with honey, if you wish, just before serving.

Asparagus Bread Pudding

Bread pudding is one of those magical concoctions whereby a few humble ingredients are slapped together and transformed into something comforting, delicious, and divine. This one's savory. SERVES 8

- 2 tablespoons olive oil or unsalted butter
- 2 small organic leeks, light parts only, cleaned well and cut into ½-inch thick slices
- 5 organic eggs
- 3 cups organic milk
- 1 pound organic asparagus, trimmed and cut into 1-inch pieces
- 1 pound dry bread torn into cubes
- ½ pound mixed cheeses
- 1½ cups chopped fresh herbs (chives, parsley, tarragon, chervil)
- Salt and freshly ground pepper to taste

1. Preheat the oven to 375°F. Over medium heat in a skillet, heat the olive oil or butter with a splash of water and braise the leeks for about 10 minutes, then remove from heat and let cool.

2. In a large bowl, combine the eggs and milk, then the rest of the ingredients and the leeks. Gently toss to combine ingredients, but don't stir so much that the bread falls apart.

3. Spread the mixture into a 4-quart baking dish, or any baking dish large enough to hold everything. You can also use a springform pan for a more elegant presentation.

4. Bake for 50 minutes, or until knife inserted in center comes out clean. Allow to cool slightly and serve.

Organic Processed Food

As noted, the national organic standards include a list of approved synthetic and prohibited nonsynthetic substances for organic production. This list is somewhat controversial: It has grown from 77 to 245 since it was created in 2002. Companies must appeal to the USDA's National Organic Standards Board every five years to keep a substance on the list, explaining why an organic alternative has not been found. The goal was to shrink the list over time, but only one item has been removed so far.

True Food seeks to minimize how much processed food you consume, whether it's organic or not. Making meals from scratch using fresh, whole foods is more nutritious and flavorful and means fewer additives of any kind.

TRUE TIP

Certified organic does not mean pesticide-free, but rather that in production and handling only approved synthetic and prohibited non-synthetic substances are used.

Healthy for You

HAPPY HENS PRODUCE HEALTHY EGGS

Grassfed/pastured hens are allowed to roam and subsist on a natural diet consisting of natural vegetation as well as insects and worms, whereas factory-farm hens are kept in confinement and fed grains and industrial feed that contain long ingredient lists filled with too many syllables. Although grassfed/pastured hens are not necessarily organic, they are much healthier and produce healthier eggs than factory-farm hens. *Mother Earth News* conducted nutrient tests on pastured eggs versus factory-farmed eggs. The results, as compared to the official USDA data for factory-farm eggs, show that eggs produced by pastured hens contain:

- ⅓ less cholesterol
- ¼ less saturated fat
- ⅔ more vitamin A
- Two times more omega-3 fatty acids
- Three times more vitamin E
- Seven times more beta-carotene

Organic Plum and Almond Tart

This ingredient list is long, and there is a tad of butter in here, but this tart is one of the yummiest organic plum experiences ever. SERVES 6

Pâte Sablée

- 2 cups unbleached all-purpose flour
- ¾ cup unrefined sugar
- 1 teaspoon salt
- 2 sticks (8 oz.) unsalted organic butter, chilled and diced
- 1 egg yolk

Frangipane

- 1 stick (4 oz.) unsalted organic butter, at room temperature
- ½ cup unrefined sugar
- 1 cup whole blanched almonds, finely ground
- 2 teaspoons unbleached all-purpose flour
- 1 teaspoon cornstarch
- 1 egg plus 1 egg white
- ½ vanilla bean, halved and scraped (or ½ tablespoon vanilla extract)
- 2 teaspoons almond extract
- 1 pound small organic plums, washed, halved and pitted
- 2 tablespoons raw sugar
- ¼ cup sliced almonds for garnish

FOR THE PÂTE SABLÉE

1. Preheat oven to 350°F. Combine flour, sugar, and salt in food processor. Add butter and pulse to pea size.

2. Add egg yolk and pulse until dough begins to clump—stop before it makes a ball.

3. Press dough into a 10-inch tart pan with removable bottom and trim top of dough. (There will be some left over.) Chill in freezer for 30 minutes.

4. Line shell with foil, fill with pie weights or dried beans. Bake tart shell at 350°F for 10 minutes. Remove foil and weights; bake 10 minutes more.

FOR THE FRANGIPANE

1. Combine butter and unrefined sugar in food processor. Add almonds and process.

2. Add flour and cornstarch, then egg and egg white. Process until smooth.

3. Add vanilla and almond extract; pulse to mix.

TO ASSEMBLE

1. Spread frangipane in tart shell.

2. Press plums on top, cut side up, in a pleasing design. Sprinkle with raw sugar.

3. Bake at 350°F for 45 minutes or until golden.

4. Remove and cool on a wire rack. Sprinkle with sliced almonds.

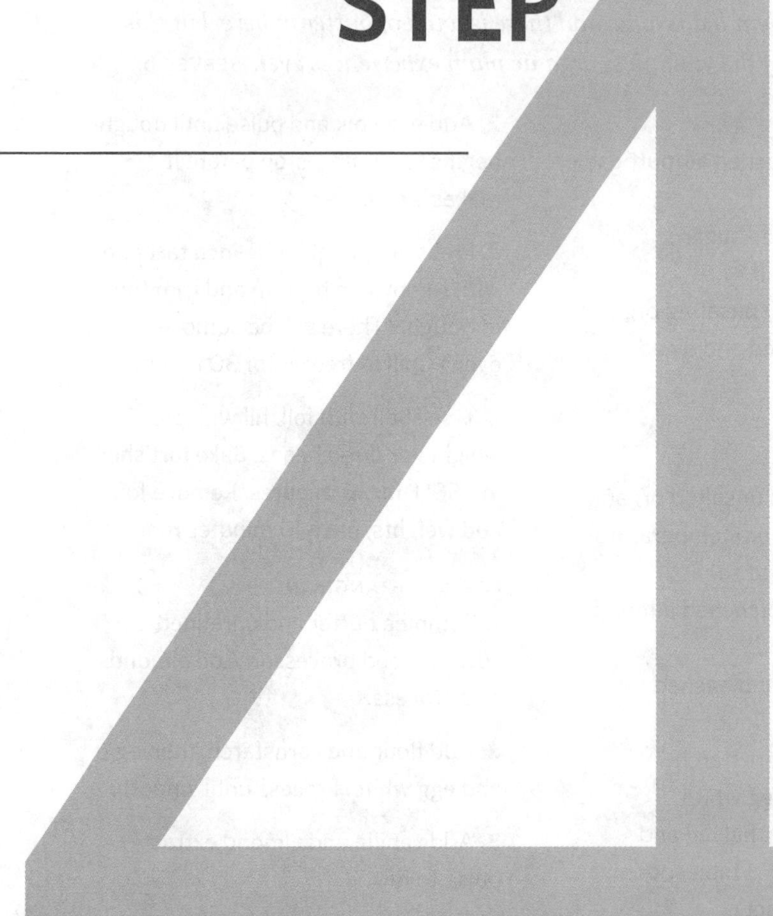

Eat Lower

ON THE FOOD CHAIN

Eating lower on the food chain means moving down a few links and becoming more of an herbivore, less of a carnivore. In short, it means eating less meat. By substituting whole grains, produce, seeds, nuts, and legumes for animal products, you reduce adverse influences on your health and on the environment. That doesn't mean you have to start eating algae and zooplankton. Just consider substituting plant-based foods for beef, pork, chicken, fish, and dairy. Doing so only three times a week can help steer your body—and the planet—in a healthier direction.

WHAT IT MEANS

The Food Chain

Going lower on the food chain means eating more whole grains, produce, and legumes.

The term "food chain" was coined in 1927 by the zoologist Charles Elton as a way to describe the interrelationships of all living things on Earth, based upon the things each species eats and in turn the species by which they are eaten.

Generally, the smallest species are at the bottom of the food chain, while larger animals are at the top. Members of each successive link eat the lower and more vulnerable species in the sequence—although nature always provides plenty of exceptions to any rule. A bird is higher on the food chain than a worm, for example, a fish higher than a fly, and a cow higher than grass. Humans can eat both high and low and be adequately nourished. Interestingly, according to scientists, foods highest on the chain are the least necessary in the human diet.

Although the American diet has tipped in favor of food choices that are high on the food chain, more and more people are starting to buck that trend. According to a 2008 study by *Vegetarian Times*, 3.2 percent of American adults (7.3 million people) follow a vegetarian-based diet. Approximately 1 million of those are vegans, who consume no animal products at all. In addition, 10 percent of American adults (22.8 million people) say their diet leans toward being vegetarian. The reasons people give: to improve their health and to save the planet.

TRUE TIP

A quick glance at nature's food chain:

On top: Carnivorous predators such as hawks, mountain lions, and humans

In the middle: Herbivores, such as cows, elephants, and deer

At the bottom: Plants and bacteria, such as zooplankton. Without them, life would not exist.

A significant part of the pleasure of eating is one's consciousness of the world from which the food comes.

—WENDELL BERRY, FARMER AND POET

How Low Can You Go?

Eating lower on the food chain can reduce the risk of disease.

Studies from around the world confirm that the lower on the food chain a human eats, the greater the protection against heart disease, cancer, and diabetes. According to the American Dietetic Association, vegetarians experience "lower mortality rates from several chronic degenerative diseases such as high blood pressure, heart disease, diabetes, and cancer, compared to non-vegetarians." Researchers present two reasons: Animal products are high in fat and lacking in fiber.

The Wrong Kind of Fat

Compared to people with high-meat diets, vegetarians have a lower death rate from heart disease. Animal products are a major source of saturated fat and cholesterol in the diet. Both increase blood levels of total cholesterol and LDL cholesterol (the bad kind) and thus increase the risk for coronary heart disease, according to the Food and Drug Administration (FDA). The National Cholesterol Education Program recommends a diet with no more than 30 percent fat and only 10 percent from saturated fat.

Chemical Concentrations

A number of chemicals created for industrial use—PCBs (insulators and coolants), PBDEs (flame retardants), dioxin (formed when chlorine-like materials are burned), and DDT, for instance—break down slowly and thus persist in the environment, lodging in the plants and animals low on the food chain. At each link up the chain, the chemical-bearing food is consumed by larger animals, the chemicals thus accumulating in higher and higher

TRUE TIP

Get your dairy fat fix with thick "sour cream" by straining plain, low-fat Greek yogurt through a colander or piece of cheesecloth over a bowl overnight.

concentrations. Consider PCBs in the food chain. Phytoplankton, the tiniest water-dwelling animals, may have a concentration of 250 parts per billion of PCBs; the herring gull, which eats the fish that ate the mysids that ate the phytoplankton, has a concentration 25 million times that. Eagles eat herring gulls, multiplying their PCB contamination 20 times again.

Humans are at the top of the food chain, and tests of body fat reveal concentrations of dioxins, PCBs, PBDEs, DDT, and other pesticides, each tied with one or more of the following: cancer, liver damage, birth defects, reproductive disorders, neurological damage, and endocrine disruption. Tragically, the chemicals DDT, dioxins, PBDEs, and PCBs not only can harm our own organs and systems but also get passed along to children in breast milk.

SNAPSHOT **MARK BITTMAN**

"I decided to do this 'vegan till 6' plan."

New York, New York

Food journalist, *New York Times*

Author, *Food Matters: A Guide to Conscious Eating with More Than 75 Recipes*

The fact is, you don't have to overhaul your eating habits totally in order to move toward true food. Consider two days a week, or a few hours a day. Like Mark Bittman. "I didn't have huge thoughts or plans about it. I just thought it was worth a try," he writes about his decision to eat lower on the food chain until 6 p.m. every day. "Within three or four months, I lost 35 pounds, my blood sugar was normal, cholesterol levels were again normal ... and my sleep apnea indeed went away. All these good things happened, and it wasn't as if I was suffering, so I stayed with it." This is not a practice of abstinence so much as changing habits. "I have not eliminated anything completely from my diet," says Bittman. A family or individual could eat lower on the food chain three days a week—and feel the difference.

WHY IT MATTERS FOR EARTH

Putting Pressure on the Environment

Reducing worldwide consumption of meat would be a step toward preserving Earth's resources.

Diets coming from lower on the food chain—largely plant-based—take less of a toll on the environment. Modern meat production involves intensive use of grain, water, energy, and grazing areas. Pork is the most resource-intensive meat, followed by beef, then poultry, eggs, and dairy products. Almost half of the energy used in American agriculture goes into livestock production.

Americans eat, on average, 67 pounds of beef and 59.2 pounds of chicken per person per year, most of it from concentrated animal feeding operations (CAFOs). The American Public Health Association has asked that states impose moratoriums on new CAFOs due to the pollution and health threats posed by factory farms.

An endocrine disruptor is any substance that behaves, when inhaled or consumed, like hormones in the endocrine system. It can interfere with reproductive processes, development, and other processes mediated by hormones.

Healthy for You

FREE RADICALS AND FAT

A good reason to reduce overall fat intake is that fats and oils promote the production of free radicals—chemicals occurring in the body that attack cells and can contribute to disease, including cancer. Oxygen causes free radicals to develop in oils. Oils rich in essential fatty acids and anti-oxidants such as vitamin E, however—such as olive oil, flaxseed oil, and fish oils—have been shown to neutralize free radicals and limit cell damage.

Seafood consumption, which hovered at around 15 pounds per capita until 2000, is expected to rise 26 percent by 2020—provided fisheries aren't depleted by overfishing.

Because most people eat a meat-based diet, the livestock population has soared, putting severe pressures on the environment, while supplies of groundwater are dwindling. Figures for how much water it takes to produce meat vary widely. The Council for Agricultural Science and Technology calculates 435 gallons for one pound of beef.

Around the world, rain forests are being deforested to make grazing land to grow soy and grain to fatten livestock. The soil beneath healthy rain forests is thin and easily destroyed after a few years of intensive grazing. Further, livestock—voracious consumers of soy and grain—consume half the world's grain harvest.

Methane production creates another environmental problem. Cows produce methane—up to 400 pounds a year. But researchers are finding that methane emission is cut by 18 percent, with no difference in milk production, when dairy cows are fed less grain and more alfalfa and flax. Industrial-scale feedlots, where tens of thousands of animals are brought into close quarters before slaughter, are also a major source of air and water pollution.

Simple Stewardship

LIVESTOCK'S LONG SHADOW

Animal farming contributes more greenhouse gases (in CO_2 equivalents, 18 percent) than all the cars, trucks, and other transportation worldwide (13.5 percent).

Water saved by one person by not eating beef for a day = 1,688 liters. Water saved by one person by not eating lamb for a day = 470 liters.

Source: Hindu Council of Australia

HOW TO DO IT

Exercise Your Options

Could you make two to three substitutions per week for meat protein in your meals?

A low-meat diet can be diverse, delicious, and nutritious, once the basics are understood. Proteins, essential to human life, are organic compounds made up of amino acids. Proteins, of course, are typically associated with eating meat. Proteins are also available from plants, but most plant foods—soy and quinoa are notable exceptions—have incomplete amino acid profiles. A combination of plant foods, such as grains and legumes, in each meal can create complete proteins.

The Facts About Fat

Almost all health professionals recommend a low-fat diet. High-fat diets increase the risk of cancer and heart disease. Yet in the panic about high-fat diets, many lump all fats together as bad. This is misleading. The American diet tends to be high in the wrong kinds of fats (from animal products and hydrogenated oils) and low in the right kinds of fats (essential fatty acids, such as the omega-3 oils). The FDA's dietary guidelines point out that some dietary fat is essential. Essential fatty acids supply energy and promote absorption of the fat-soluble vitamins A, D, E, and K.

SATURATED FAT The Dietary Guidelines for Americans state that "saturated fat raises blood cholesterol more than other forms of fat." An abundance of authoritative studies link diets high in saturated fat and cholesterol with the risk of heart disease. All animal products contain saturated fat, whereas few vegetable oils do. (Tropical plants such as avocado, peanuts, and coconut are the

TRUE TIP

Many grains are packed with protein. Quinoa is as versatile as rice but has a higher protein content than most grains because it contains all the essential amino acids.

exceptions—containing around 18 to 20 percent saturated fat.) Canola oil contains the lowest saturated fat concentration, at 6 percent.

Saturated fat—butter being the perfect example—is solid at room temperature. While the Dietary Guidelines recommend less than 30 percent of calories from fat, they also recommend only 10 percent of calories should come from saturated fat— meaning that the rest of your calories from fat should come from unsaturated fats. Ways to reduce your intake of saturated fat include cutting back on meat and choosing low-fat or skim milk.

UNSATURATED FATS Less stable than saturated fats, unsaturated fats remain liquid at room temperature. Unsaturated fats—those with the lowest concentrations of saturated fats—include canola, safflower, and flaxseed.

MONO- AND POLYUNSATURATED FATS Both mono- and polyunsaturated fats and oils are linked to reducing serum cholesterol. Some studies suggest that monounsaturated oils, while lowering "bad" cholesterol, don't reduce HDL (high-density lipoprotein), or "good" cholesterol—hence olive and canola oils' claim to fame.

Healthy for You

HOW MUCH FAT IS OK?

Current guidelines recommend obtaining less that 30 percent of calories from fat. Many health practitioners believe that number should be even lower, closer to 10 or 20 percent. (Most Americans get 40 percent of their calories from fat.) Equally important is what kind of fats you consume.

Healthy for You

COMBOS FOR A FULL PROTEIN

Our bodies are made up of 22 amino acids, 8 of which we cannot synthesize and must get from outside sources. Every single one of these 22 amino acids must be present at the same time in order for the body to synthesize protein.

The missing 8 are called the "limiting amino acids," and they must be present not only at the same time but also in the right proportions. They are: valine, leucine, and isoleucine, the sulfur-containing amino acids; methionine, an aromatic amino acid; and phenylalanine, tryptophan, threonine, and lysine. For If you combine certain foods that have these complementary amino acids, such as legumes and a grain, you can make a full protein.

Even if you ingest all of the amino acids, not all of the protein from food is used by our bodies. Net protein utilization (NPU) is the percentage of ingested protein in a given food item the body actually uses. An egg is the ideal protein with 94 percent NPU; milk is nearly as good.

COMPLEMENTARY PROTEIN COMBINATIONS

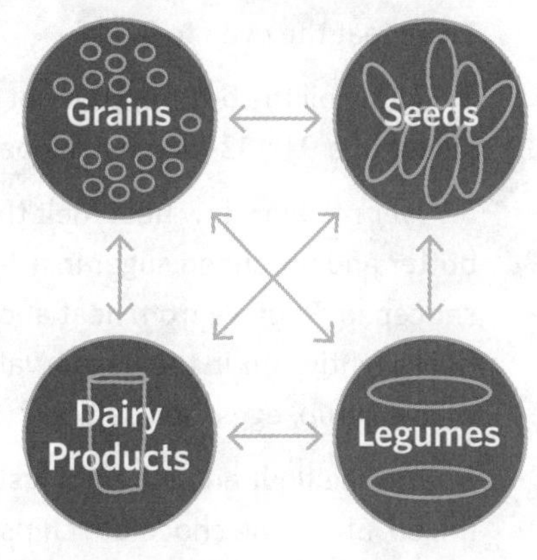

FOOD	NPU
most meats	57-65%
eggs	94%
milk	82%
soybeans (alone)	61%
other legumes alone	50-60%
brown rice	70%
other whole grains	50-60%

source: *Diet for a Small Planet*

Nothing will benefit human health and increase chances for survival of life on Earth as much as the evolution to a vegetarian diet. —ALBERT EINSTEIN

(Olive oil has 82 percent monounsaturates, canola has 60 percent.) Other unrefined oils relatively high in monounsaturated fats include almond, peanut, pistachio, pecan, canola, avocado, hazelnut, cashew, and macadamia.

Unrefined polyunsaturated oils are high in omega-6, and include safflower oil (79 percent polyunsaturated), sunflower oil (60 percent), corn oil (60 percent), and soy oil (50 percent). Don't mistake trans-polyunsaturated (hydrogenated and partially hydrogenated) oils for acceptable oils, because they can interfere with the metabolism of essential fatty acids.

White Bean Blondies

Brownies, blondies, cookies, fresh from the oven—and all that butter, refined flour, and sugar. But here's an alternative. This recipe substitutes white beans, halves the animal fat, and boosts the protein. MAKES 24

- 8 tablespoons unsalted organic butter
- ½ cup unrefined sugar
- 1½ cups pureed white beans
- 1 teaspoon pure vanilla extract
- ½ cup maple syrup
- 2 large eggs
- ½ teaspoon salt
- 1¾ cup white whole wheat flour
- 1 cup chocolate chips, optional

1. Preheat the oven to 325°F.

2. Lightly oil the bottom (but not the sides) of a 9 by 13-inch baking pan.

3. Over medium-low heat melt the butter and unrefined sugar in a saucepan. Remove from heat and let cool slightly. Stir in the beans, vanilla, maple syrup, eggs, and salt.

4. Add the flour and stir until just mixed. Stir in the chocolate chips if you're using them, then pour the entire mixture into the prepared baking pan.

5. Bake for 30 to 33 minutes, until a tester comes out clean. Allow to cool completely in the pan before cutting.

Healthy for You

EAT THE RIGHT KIND OF FATS

The FDA's dietary guidelines point out that some dietary fat is essential. But the dietary fats they are talking about—essential fatty acids—come from plants.

Essential fatty acids are omega-3 and omega-6, two oil molecules that the body cannot make for itself. Crucial for life and well-being, these essential fatty acids are available in some foods. Omega-3 oils can be found in pumpkin, canola, wheat germ, rice bran, flax (linseed oil), walnuts, and soy. Omega-6 oils are found in all vegetable oils, particularly safflower, sunflower, corn, and sesame oils. Many nutritionists believe that omega-3 oils are the least consumed of the fats—and therefore the ones that most of us are likely to be deficient in.

Essential fatty acids supply energy and promote absorption of the fat-soluble vitamins A, D, E, and K. Cholesterol is found only in animal products, and saturated fat is found primarily in animal products.

Symptoms of fatty acid deficiency include dry skin, lusterless hair, soft fingernails that break easily, and little raised "goose bumps" on the back of the arms and sometimes the thighs. These fats can even affect mood: A recent study from the National Institute on Alcohol Abuse and Alcoholism links omega-3 deficiency to increased depression and aggression.

SUPERUNSATURATED OILS Superunsaturated oils are excellent choices because they are high in omega-3. Flax oil is by far the highest source at 57 percent superunsaturated, followed by pumpkin seed oil (15 percent), canola oil (10 percent), soy oil (8 percent), and walnut oil (5 percent).

TRANS-FATTY ACIDS In the rush to replace solid, spreadable butter, which is full of saturated fat and cholesterol, scientists came up with a process called hydrogenation. Hydrogenated and partially hydrogenated fats are made up of unsaturated fats, but they are artificially hardened; margarine and shortening are the most common examples. Advertised as containing no cholesterol or saturated fat, hydrogenated oils once seemed to be the answer for those concerned about heart disease.

But now concerns have surfaced about the havoc trans-fatty acids may wreak in the body, including atherosclerosis and cancer. One serious problem is that if too many trans-fatty acids are ingested, they interfere with essential fatty acid function. Given that many Americans may be borderline deficient in omega-3 oils to begin with, interfering with their ability to function is not recommended for optimum health.

On January 1, 2008, the FDA mandated that manufacturers are required to list trans fat on the Nutrition Facts panel of foods and some dietary supplements. Read labels carefully, but note that trans-fat levels of less than 0.5

Pumpkin Seed Pesto

Hulled pumpkin seeds, also known as pepitos, are high in protein, iron, and minerals. Use them in pesto, with just about any combination of fresh herbs, to "meaten" up your meatless pasta dishes. Serve this mixed with pasta and topped with extra pumpkin seeds.

- ½ cup pumpkin seeds, hulled and roasted, plus more for garnish
- 2 tablespoons grated Parmesan cheese or roasted cashews
- 1 garlic clove
- 1½ cups (total) parsley, basil, cilantro, or other herbs of choice
- 2 teaspoons lemon juice
- ⅓ cup extra-virgin olive oil or pumpkin seed oil
- Salt and pepper to taste

1. Place pumpkin seeds, cheese or cashews, and garlic in a food processor with the metal blade. Process until mixture is ground, about 30 seconds.

2. Add herbs and lemon juice. Pulse, and slowly add olive oil until the mixture is finely chopped and olive oil is just blended in. Taste and season.

SNAPSHOT **SIDNEY BAKER**

"A deficiency of the essential fatty acid supplied by the omega-3 oils is epidemic."

Sag Harbor, New York

Environmental health pioneer

Author, *Detoxification & Healing*

How could anyone in our society have a deficiency of fat? Sidney Baker believes one reason for this epidemic is a change in the processing of vegetable oils, which began around 1950. Essential fatty acids were actually removed from oils in the interest of extending shelf life. Saturated oils, such as corn, palm, peanut, safflower, and sunflower oils, are preferred by manufacturers because their shelf life is longer. This tradeoff of omega-3 oils for longer shelf life, along with the widespread distribution of vegetable oils, says Baker, has resulted in an imbalance in oils that we need to produce healthy cell membranes.

grams per serving can be listed as 0 grams trans fat on the food label.

Vegetarian Diets

People may choose to become vegetarian and stop eating meat products altogether to avoid "bad" fats. There are 12.5 million vegetarians in the United States at present, and the number is growing. A lacto-ovo vegetarian eats dairy products and eggs, a lacto-vegetarian eats dairy foods but no eggs, and a vegan eats no animal foods of any kind.

Does your city ban trans fats in restaurants? If not, work to make it happen! Health problems associated with trans fats are so serious that The American Medical Association supports the ban of artificial trans fats in U.S. restaurants and bakeries.

VITAMIN B_{12} AND THE VEGAN DIET In the new Dietary Guidelines for Americans, the USDA and Department of Health and Human Services advise that vegans supplement their diets with B_{12} by taking supplements. The only proven source of vitamin B_{12} is animal products, and the American Dietetic Association does not believe that spirulina, seaweed, and tempeh and other fermented foods are reliable sources of vitamin B_{12}. Two other nutritional concerns for vegans, especially children, are vitamin D and calcium, both found in milk. (Vitamin D is added to milk by most dairies.)

When You Eat High on the Food Chain

Ninety percent of Americans eat animal products. There are ways to choose among meat products to find those healthiest for us and for the environment. There are a number of other ways to support sustainable farming

Cooking & Eating

EXPLORE NEW FOODS

Soy can be a simple solution for a meat substitute, given how easy it is to use tofu or "faux meats" made of soy. But relying too much on a single type of protein can lead to food allergies.

Another common pitfall for new vegetarians is to depend on dairy products, especially cheese, for protein. Although cheese is fine in moderation, it is high in fat. And dairy products, higher on the food chain, can contain fat contaminated with pesticides, PCBs, and dioxin.

Vegetarians should eat an adequate quantity and variety of food to get proper amounts of protein, iron, zinc, and B vitamins, typically found in higher amounts in meat, poultry, and fish.

Try these high-protein vegetarian alternatives:

- Beans in tacos and tostadas
- Bean patties, veggie burgers
- Protein-packed pumpkin seeds or sunflower seeds in salads and pasta, or as a snack
- Nut butters: almond, cashew, macadamia, hempseed
- Vegetarian lentil or split pea soup—protein powerhouses

practices, such as buying from farms that are certified for treating animals humanely, practicing habitat protection, and working to protect watersheds.

In general, the best choices are free-range meats or poultry fed organic feed and raised on a sustainable farm without antibiotics or growth stimulants.

Maple Vanilla Horchata

Horchata is a delicious alternative to cow's milk. It originated in Spain and typically includes rice, almonds, sugar, and cinnamon. Our nutritious version uses brown rice and maple syrup and a whole vanilla bean to round out the flavor. SERVES 8 TO 10

1 cup long-grain brown rice
2 cups whole almonds
1 vanilla bean
8 cups water
½ cup maple syrup

1. Rinse and drain the rice.

2. Use a spice (or coffee) grinder to grind the rice until fine.

3. Combine the rice with the almonds in a large bowl. Split the vanilla bean and scrape into the rice, then drop the whole bean in. Pour in 3 ½ cups of water, cover, and let sit overnight.

4. Remove the vanilla bean from the rice mixture, then pour the mixture into a blender and blend until smooth. Add 2 ½ cups of water and continue blending. Add maple syrup.

5. Strain horchata with a metal strainer, and then strain again using a double layer of cheesecloth.

6. Add up to an additional 2 cups of water until it gets to the consistency you like.

How to Choose the Best Beef

Meat eaters looking for healthier, tastier beef have a range of options these days, but how does one distinguish a grassfed cow from a humanely raised cow? The best labels have detailed and specific standards that leave little room for loopholes. We've examined six of the most common labels on the shelf of your local grocer and determined how they stack up in terms of feed, access to pasture, antibiotics, growth hormones, and animal welfare. Though many responsible farmers go above and beyond a label's requirements, the American Grassfed Association's labels provide the most green guarantees across the widest array of issues.

TRUE TIP

Flour Power! Boost protein by thinking outside of the flour box. High-protein flours include quinoa, bran, soy, spelt, and garbanzo.

Healthy for You

CHECK FOR HIGH-NUTRIENT FOODS

When eating lower on the food chain, pay particular attention to foods rich in zinc, calcium, B_{12}, and iron. If you eat a varied diet, you should be getting all the nutrients you need.

The Asian Food Pyramid recommends eating fruits, legumes, nuts and seeds, vegetables, and grains daily.

Nuts and seeds are high in the mineral zinc, as are beans and whole grains.

Beans, nuts and seeds, seaweeds, whole grains, and some fruits, such as raisins and watermelon, are high in iron.

B_{12} is the only vitamin available only in animal products and must be supplemented.

Calcium is widely available in dairy products, in tofu (if processed with calcium sulfate), and in dark green leafy vegetables such as kale, mustard greens, and turnip greens.

Vitamin D is synthesized by the body when a person is exposed to the sun. Most modern humans don't make enough. Light-skinned people need about 15 minutes of sun a day for adequate vitamin D synthesis; dark-skinned people need twice that.

Cooking & Eating

THE SECRETS OF SAUCES

A key to making vegan and vegetarian meals interesting is to develop four or five favorite sauces that can easily be adapted for legumes, the animal-free protein mainstay. In *The Art of Simple Food,* Alice Waters provides four sauces— aioli, salsa verde, herbed butter, and a vinaigrette—and though they are basic, they add flavor, dimension, and color to meals. Any one of them can pull a meal together and help you turn a simple plate of legumes and vegetables into a finished dish. And they're so easy to prepare that once you've made them a few times, you'll never have to look up the recipes again. Another great resource that offers 500 simple and flavorful sauce recipes is *Get Saucy* by Grace Parisi.

Black Bean Hummus

Hummus is a gift! A quick, rich, creamy dish packed with protein and devoid of animal fat. Use a variety of beans to create different tastes. This recipe uses black beans, lime, and cilantro for an earthy taste—and a change of pace from traditional hummus. Serve with toasted pita triangles or vegetables, or in sandwiches.

- 2 cups cooked black beans, drained
- ¼ cup tahini
- 2 teaspoons lime juice
- 1½ tablespoons olive oil
- 1 minced garlic clove
- 1 teaspoon ground cumin
- ½ cup chopped cilantro
- ¼ teaspoon cayenne pepper

Make sure the beans are drained well and rinsed. Combine all ingredients in food processor and combine until smooth, adding more lime juice and olive oil to thin the hummus as needed.

TYPE OF FEED USED Compared with grain- and corn-fed beef, grassfed beef packs a higher nutritional punch and has less fat, less cholesterol, and fewer calories than corn- and grain-fed beef. Grassfed beef also has higher concentrations of vitamin E, beta-carotene, vitamin C, and omega-3 fatty acids. For livestock health, grass is the best feed. Corn- and grain-based diets also can lead to high levels of *E. coli* bacteria among the animals.

ACCESS TO PASTURE This phrase is commonly used to imply that cattle spent the majority of their time

---

Nut Milks Two Ways

Nondairy milks are great for people who are lactose intolerant or vegan and for those looking to eat lower on the food chain. An increasing number of commercial nut milks are becoming widely available, but many are highly processed or use surprising ingredients. It is easy to make a nonprocessed version at home. Here are two methods—add a tablespoon of coconut butter to either for a richer result.

Almost Instant Nut Milk

- 2 tablespoons of your favorite nut butter
- 2 cups water
- Pinch of sea salt
- 2 tablespoons honey
- ½ teaspoon vanilla extract

Blend all ingredients in a blender until smooth.

Basic Nut Milk

- 1 cup raw almonds, soaked in water for at least 4 hours
- 3 cups water
- Optionally, add: dates, banana, vanilla extract, sea salt, maple syrup

After the nuts have soaked, blenderize nuts and water for about 2 minutes.

Strain the mix twice through multiple layers of cheesecloth placed in a colander or sieve.

Fun, Kids, Pleasure

PLANT-BASED PROTEIN POWER

Tell your kids that plant protein gives them superpowers. Try these fun alternatives to chicken nuggets and hot dogs.

- **EDAMAME** This great source of protein is easy on young palates and fun to pop and eat.
- **TRAIL MIX** Make your own nut and fruit mixes with your kids' favorites.
- **BURRITO BAR** Set out bowls of cooked beans, rice or other grains, sliced avocado, tomatoes, lettuce, steamed vegetables, and a basket of warmed whole-grain tortillas, for roll-your-own burritos.
- **SLOW-ROASTED TOFU** Cut into thin slices, coat lightly with olive oil, and roast slowly.

outdoors. For some labels, "access" isn't clearly defined; an animal that spends only a little time on the range can be certified as having "access to pasture." To avoid ambiguity, look for labels that give more specific requirements than "access to pasture."

ANTIBIOTICS Forty percent of the antibiotics sold in the United States are used in agriculture, largely for feed additives given to cattle to promote growth. This practice has sent chemicals into our waterways and caused physical changes in aquatic life. The overuse of antibiotics in livestock has also contributed to a rise in drug-resistant bacteria in humans.

GROWTH HORMONES Two-thirds of the beef cattle raised in the U.S. each year receive growth hormones. Though only trace amounts of the hormones are found in the end meat product, hormonally charged agricultural runoff has

Beef Labels

	USDA ORGANIC*	USDA GRASS-FED	AMERICAN GRASSFED ASSOCIATION
Feed	• 100% organic grass • 100% organic corn • 100% organic grain	• Grass (If an animal consumes a prohibited feed source, the farmer must document the type, the amount, and the frequency, but the end product can still bear the USDA Grass-fed label.)	• Grass only
Access to Pasture	Required, but "access" is not clearly defined.	Required, but "access" is not clearly defined.	Required standards ensure that animals spend the majority of their lives on pasture.
Antibiotics	Given only to sick animals, which are then removed from the program.	Allowed	Given only to sick animals, which are then removed from the program.
Growth Hormones	None allowed	Allowed	None allowed
Animal Welfare	Vague criteria	Not addressed	Vague criteria

* After processing, beef products containing only organic ingredients can be labeled "100% organic." Products containing 95-100% organic ingredients can be labeled "organic."

** Only family farms are eligible for certification by the Animal Welfare Institute.

***The Food Alliance Label also guarantees that cattle have been slaughtered humanely.

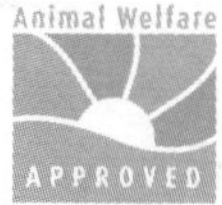 **ANIMAL WELFARE APPROVED****	CERTIFIED HUMANE RAISED & HANDLED **CERTIFIED HUMANE RASIED AND HANDLED**	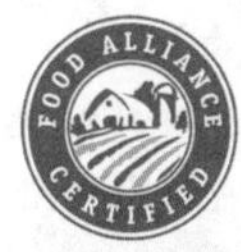 **FOOD ALLIANCE CERTIFIED*****
• Corn • Grass • Grain	• Corn • Grass • Grain	• Corn • Grass • Grain • Animal protein
Required standards ensure that animals spend the majority of their lives on pasture.	Not required	Required standards ensure that animals spend the majority of their lives on pasture.
Given only to sick animals.	Given only to sick animals.	Given only to sick animals.
None allowed	None allowed	None allowed
Very specific requirements addressing a variety of issues, including health, shelter, and handling.	Very specific requirements addressing a variety of issues, including health, shelter, and handling.	Very specific requirements addressing a variety of issues, including health, shelter, and handling.

been found to threaten the reproductive capabilities of fish in U.S. waterways.

Never buy imported shellfish. The risk of bacterial contamination is too great, due to poor handling and irregular refrigeration practices. Ask your grocer where all seafood comes from.

ANIMAL WELFARE Inhumane treatment of animals is detrimental not only to cattle but also to consumers who eat the beef. Maltreated, sick cows may pass on diseases to beef products, and the waste of diseased cattle can pollute streams and waterways near farms and plants. The more rigorous labels provide detailed rules that ensure animal health and clean, comfortable

Shopping & Saving

COMPARE THE COST PER POUND

ORGANIC PUMPKIN SEEDS
bulk: $4.29*
packaged: $7.99
Almost 2x cheaper to buy bulk

ORGANIC SUNFLOWER SEEDS
bulk: $2.99*
packaged: $4.99
1.7x cheaper to buy bulk

ORGANIC OATS
bulk: $1.19*
packaged: $4.09 *
3.5x cheaper to buy bulk

ORGANIC QUINOA
bulk: $3.99*
packaged: $6.84*
1.7x cheaper to buy bulk

* Prices as of June 2009 in Rhinebeck, NY

ORGANIC PINTO BEANS
bulk: $2.15*
canned: $2.66*
1.25x cheaper to buy bulk

ORGANIC BLACK-EYED PEAS
bulk: $1.99
packaged: $2.15
canned: $2.49
bulk 1.1x cheaper than packaged
bulk 1.25x cheaper than canned

HAMBURGER TACOS VERSUS BEAN TACOS
beans: $1.00 a pound*
antibiotic-free hamburger: $4.99 a pound*

90-percent fat-free hamburger: $4.79 a pound*
Beans are about 1/5 the price of hamburger.

environments; they also require producers to manage cattle so as to reduce stress to the animals and limit painful techniques, such as branding and electric prodding.

Fish and Shellfish

Fish and shellfish provide lean protein with great health benefits, but sometimes fish can be bad for you, and some fishing practices can be bad for the environment. Seafood can be contaminated with high levels of mercury and PCBs, causing ill health effects. Pollution and habitat destruction of the marine environment lead to the loss of several million tons of edible fish a year. Fish can accumulate fat-soluble pesticides like DDT, industrial chemicals like PCBs and dioxins, and toxic metals like mercury in their systems. Clams and oysters can accumulate lead and cadmium. Children and pregnant women are the most at risk.

Fried Tilapia (or Lake Perch)

Here is a simple, flavorful recipe created by Will Allen of Milwaukee's Growing Power National Training and Community Food Center. It uses tilapia, one of the safest and most environmentally friendly fish to eat.

SERVES 2 TO 6

1 fish, 1 to 1½ pounds, per person
6 eggs
1 cup milk
Flour and cornmeal or bread crumbs
Canola oil

1. Mix eggs and milk in a large bowl.

2. Soak fish in egg and milk batter for 10 to 15 minutes.

3. Mix flour and cornmeal in equal portions. (For extra crispiness, use flour and bread crumbs—or all three.)

4. Roll fish in flour-cornmeal mix. Gently shake off excess.

5. Heat ½ inch of canola oil in a large castiron skillet.

6. Fry fish on medium heat for 10 minutes, 5 minutes on each side.

Simple Stewardship

CONSUMER'S GUIDE TO MERCURY

The list below shows the amount of various types of fish that a woman who is pregnant or planning to become pregnant can safely eat, according to the Environmental Protection Agency (EPA). People with small children who want to use the list as a guide should reduce portion sizes. Adult men, and women who are not planning to become pregnant, are less at risk from mercury exposure but may wish to refer to the list for low-mercury choices.

Protecting yourself —and the fish

Certain fish, even some low in mercury, are poor choices for other reasons, most often because they have been overfished so extensively that their numbers are perilously low. These fish are marked with an asterisk (read more below).

This list applies to fish caught and sold commercially. For information about fish you catch yourself, check for advisories in your state.

Least Mercury

Enjoy these fish:

Anchovies
Butterfish
Catfish
Clams
Crab (Domestic)
Crawfish/Crayfish
Croaker (Atlantic)
Flounder*
Haddock (Atlantic)*
Hake
Herring
Mackerel (N. Atlantic, Chub)
Mullet
Oysters
Perch (Ocean)
Plaice
Pollock
Salmon (Canned)**
Salmon (Fresh)**
Sardines
Scallops*
Shad (American)
Shrimp*
Sole (Pacific)
Squid (Calamari)
Tilapia
Trout (Freshwater)
Whitefish
Whiting

IN FISH (AND TO OVER-FISHED SPECIES)

Moderate Mercury

Eat six servings or less per month:

Bass (Striped, Black)
Carp
Cod (Alaskan)*
Croaker (White Pacific)
Halibut (Atlantic)*
Halibut (Pacific)
Jacksmelt (Silverside)
Lobster
Mahi Mahi
Monkfish*
Perch (Freshwater)
Sablefish
Skate*
Snapper*
Tuna (Canned chunk light)
Tuna (Skipjack)*
Weakfish (Sea Trout)
Weakfish (Sea Trout)

High Mercury

Eat three servings or less per month:

Bluefish
Grouper*
Mackerel (Spanish, Gulf)
Sea Bass (Chilean)*
Tuna (Canned Albacore)
Tuna (Yellowfin)*

Highest Mercury

Avoid eating:

Mackerel (King)
Marlin*
Orange Roughy*
Shark*
Swordfish*
Tilefish*
Tuna (Bigeye, Ahi)*

* **Fish in trouble!** These fish are perilously low in numbers or are caught by environmentally destructive methods.

** **Farmed salmon** may contain PCBs, chemicals with serious long-term health effects. Select only organic farmed salmon.

The data for this guide come from the U.S. Food and Drug Administration, which tests fish for mercury, and the U.S. Environmental Protection Agency, which determines safe mercury levels for women of childbearing age.

Mercury-level categories represent the following in the flesh of tested fish:

Least mercury: Less than 0.09 parts per million

Moderate mercury: From 0.09 to 0.29 pppm

High mercury: From 0.3 to 0.49 ppm

Highest mercury: More than 0.5 ppm

Source: National Resources Defense Council

For up-to-date information on fish choices for health and the environment, visit these websites: Monterey Bay Aquarium *(www.montereybayaquarium.org/cr/seafoodwatch.aspx)* and the Blue Ocean Institute *(www.blueocean.org/seafood/seafood-guide)*.

STEP

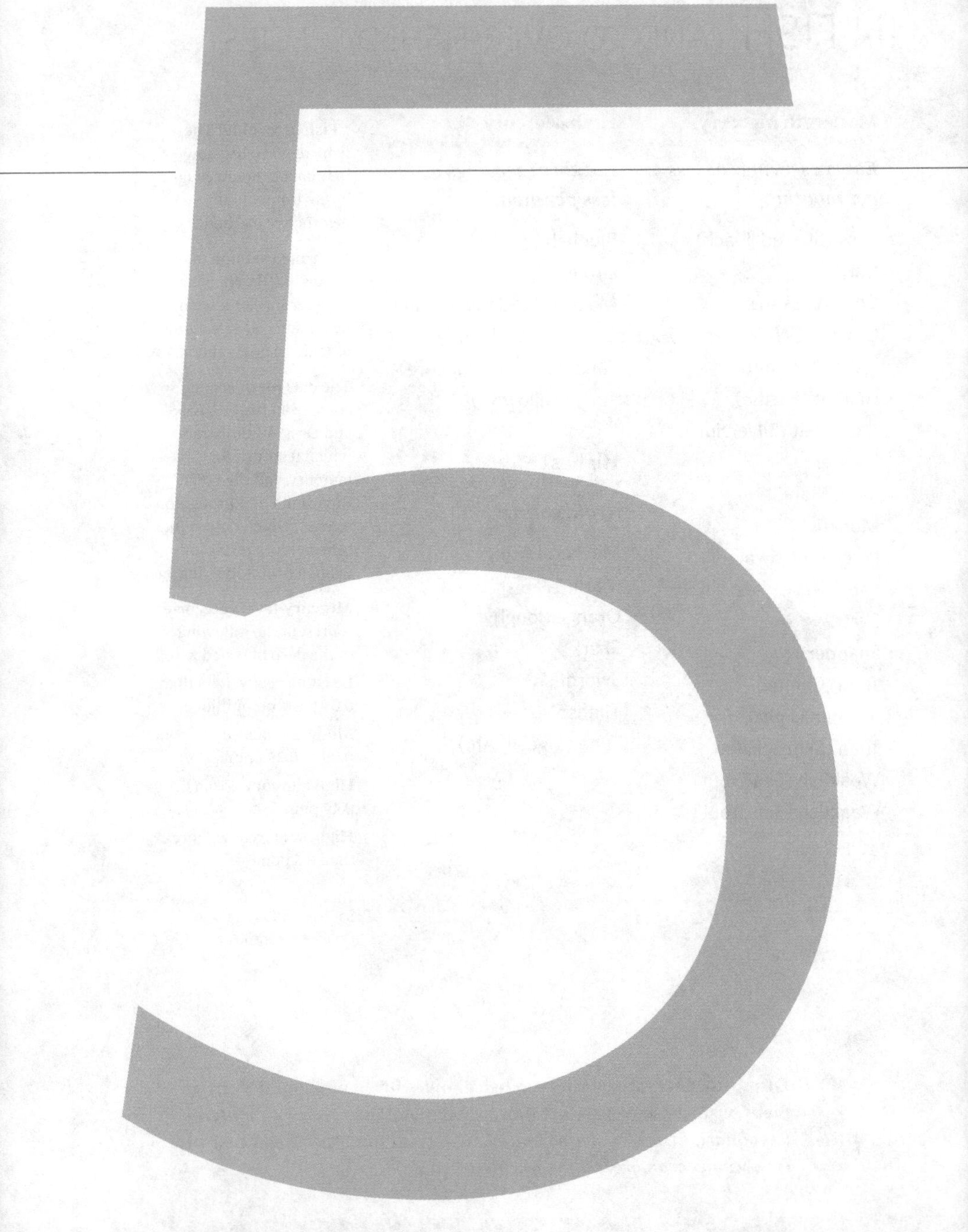

Eat Fresh Food

Eating fresh food is eating true food. And just what, you might ask, is true food? It is food made from seeds, soil, sunlight, and water—not chemicals, conveyor belts, and seductive marketing. It's food that came out of the ground and found its way to your plate with as little interference as possible. True fresh food actually resembles what it looked like in the field and is alive with the flavors of nature.

WHAT IT MEANS

Fresh Food

Fresh food, living food, food that was recently alive on Earth—this choice is central to good eating.

What does it mean to eat fresh food? For nutrition educator Joan Gussow, it means to "just eat food." For nutritionist John Yudkin, it means not eating "anything your Neolithic ancestors wouldn't have recognized." (Or, adds author Michael Pollan, your great-grandmother.) Eating fresh food is as simple as it sounds—it doesn't mean avoiding all canned, dried, and frozen food, which many of us rely on when eating seasonally, but rather, eating produce as close to its natural state as possible—and within a reasonable time from its harvest. We could just as easily say eat living food. For those dedicated to a raw food diet, living food means food not heated beyond 116°F. We define living or fresh food as food that hasn't been compromised by the addition of preservatives, transformed into a food product by additives, or created by food scientists in a lab.

WHY IT MATTERS FOR YOU

Fresh Does Mean Better

Foods transformed into "food products" means more fat and fewer nutrients.

Some 17,000 new food products (things that Michael Pollan prefers to call "foodlike substitutes") are introduced annually to the market. Produce is transformed into products filled with preservatives, sweeteners, fat, and salt—thus decimating the enzymes, fiber, and micronutrients in fresh food.

Take a product like potato crisps—made from dried potatoes and extruded in an identical shape. Calorie for calorie, most potato crisps have nine and a half times the salt, nine times the fat, 75 percent less fiber and protein, and none of the recommended daily allowances for iron and calcium, compared to a fresh, whole potato. (Interesting that it was fantasy and science fiction writer Gene Wolfe who developed the machine that cooks the leading brand of potato crisps!)

In terms of eating food as soon after harvest as possible, consider this. Uncooked vegetables can lose from 10 to 50 percent of their less stable nutrients in two weeks—which, given the current food system, can be the very length of time it takes to get food from a large-scale commercial farm to your table.

WHY IT MATTERS FOR EARTH

Processing and Polluting

Food-processing industries leave a trail of organic and inorganic waste.

Wastewater and solid wastes are the primary causes of pollution concern within the fruit and vegetable food-processing industry. Wastewater from processing plants is high in suspended solids, organic sugars, and starches, and may contain residual pesticides. Solid wastes contain organic materials from mechanical preparation processes, including rinds, seeds, and skins from raw materials. All of this amounts to more reasons to find your produce locally, because local fruits and vegetables have not traveled through the industrial processing plants on their way to your kitchen.

The primary steps in processing fresh fruits and fresh vegetables for safe eating and storage include:

- General cleaning and dirt removal
- Removal of leaves, skin, and seeds
- Blanching
- Washing and cooling
- Packaging
- Cleanup

SNAPSHOT **JOY ALAIDAROUS**

"Since eating only fresh and all natural foods, I've gained more vitality and feel like the bodily aging process has slowed way down."

Pasadena, California

School psychologist

In 2001 Joy Alaidarous discovered that she had developed a severe intolerance to anything containing the slightest trace of soy. And although she pored over food labels, she found that soy is used so widely in processed food, an innocent-sounding ingredient such as "natural flavor" or "emulsifier" could give her a debilitating three-day migraine because it contained soy. Her solution? She stopped eating processed food altogether. She no longer has migraines, her cholesterol levels and weight have dropped, her health has improved, and she feels lively and vibrant. How did she do it? She moved to a bigger backyard and created a vegetable garden. She bought a number of vegetarian cookbooks. She shops at her local farmers' market and on the perimeters of the supermarket, rarely venturing into the center aisles, where processed food is shelved. She takes her lunch to work and eats out only at restaurants where the kitchen uses fresh ingredients. And she always offers to bring a dish to a dinner or party, so there will be at least one thing she can eat!

One of the problems with the food processing industry's use and discharge of large amounts of water is that it takes place in rural areas where the potable water and wastewater systems are designed to serve small populations. As a result, one medium-size plant can have a major effect on local water supply and surface water quality. Large food-processing plants typically use more than a million gallons of potable water per day. Other primary issues of concern include both organic and packaging waste. Organic waste—that is, the rinds, seeds, and skins from raw materials—results from processing operations. Inorganic waste typically includes excessive packaging made of plastic, glass, and metal.

HOW TO DO IT

Strive for Five—and More

Eat as much fresh food—vegetables, fruits, and nuts—as possible.

The National Cancer Institute recommends that each of us eats at least five servings of fresh fruits and vegetables a day, since the complex carbohydrates and fiber they contain play a very beneficial role in protecting against cancer, heart disease, and common digestive ailments. Many nutritionists recommend nine to ten servings of fruits and vegetables a day.

If you spread at least five servings of fruit and vegetables out over three meals a day plus snacks, reaching the goal of five servings a day isn't so hard, even for a child. If you eat a vegetable at lunch and dinner, and fruit at two meals and a snack, you'll be all set. If you are unable to have a vegetable at lunch, you can have a salad and a vegetable at dinner.

Eat More Nuts and Seeds

Because of their fat content, nuts and seeds are often mistakenly relegated to the list of foods one should never eat. But there is a lot about nuts that is worthy of attention. Studies have shown that those who consume nuts regularly have a lower rate of heart attack or coronary death compared with those who eat them rarely.

Nuts and seeds are a rich source of essential fatty acids such as omega-3 oils, known to boost heart health. Of course that means that they are high in fat, although most nuts and seeds are high in monounsaturated and polyunsaturated fats, low in saturated fats, and cholesterol-free. Chestnuts are the least fatty, with 13 percent of calories from fat, whereas coconut and macadamia nuts get 88 percent and 95 percent, respectively, of their calories from fat.

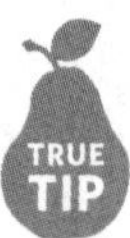

Caution: Aflatoxin, a mold that grows on peanuts, is carcinogenic. The Valencia peanut grows in drier climates and is less likely to have aflatoxin contamination.

Green Pea, Mint, and Pistachio Pesto

Many of us will never, ever get tired of traditional basil pesto—but if there are peas around and plenty of mint in your garden (or at the market), nothing beats this pesto. Toss it with pasta, stir it into rice, smear it on a toasted baguette, or use it to top poached fish.

- 2 cups fresh peas
- ½ cup pistachio nuts
- 1 garlic clove
- ¼ cup mint leaves
- ½ cup grated Parmesan cheese
- ⅓ cup olive oil
- ½ teaspoon salt
- Freshly ground pepper

1. Set aside some peas, pistachios, and a few mint leaves for garnish.

2. With food processor running, drop in garlic and finely chop. Next add peas, pistachios, mint, cheese, salt, and pepper, and process until finely chopped. Keep motor running and add oil until combined.

Toss pesto with cooked pasta and garnish with reserved peas, pistachios, and mint. Serve warm or cold.

Nuts and seeds are also rich in zinc and iron. Next to sea vegetables, they have some of the highest mineral content of any plant food. The USDA Food Pyramid classifies them as protein, but they must be complemented by other plant proteins in a vegetarian diet. Other than legumes, they are the only protein source that also contains fiber.

Buy pecans in dull brown shells; shiny, reddish shells have been dyed. Many pistachios are artificially dyed white or red as well. To avoid dyes, buy shelled nuts in health food stores.

HOW TO BUY AND STORE NUTS Make sure nuts are fresh, and avoid any that are discolored, shriveled, rubbery, obviously moldy, or taste stale. If you buy nuts in bulk, ask the store for permission to taste a sample before buying in quantity. It is the oil in nuts that goes rancid.

- Buy organic nuts if possible, since high-fat foods (like nuts) have greater concentrations of pesticides.
- Blanched nuts may be chemically processed.
- Buy nuts in the shell because they are the freshest and keep the longest. Refrigerate them in an airtight glass jar for up to three months, longer in the freezer.
- Buy nuts during the fall harvest and freeze them. Whole nuts keep longer than broken bits.
- Light makes free radicals in oils, so store nuts in a dark place. When the oils in nuts go rancid, the nuts should not be eaten.

NUT BUTTERS Freshly ground nut butters are incomparably more flavorful than those from jars. You can buy them in a store that grinds them on the spot, or you can grind your own at home, using a food processor or grinder.

When buying commercial nut butters, avoid those made with partially hydrogenated oils. Unopened nut butters have a shelf life of six to nine months. Opened nut butters should be stored in the refrigerator and will last about two weeks.

STEP 5 | EAT FRESH FOOD

Guide to Nuts and Seeds

Almonds (Sweet)

Flavorful nut grown widely in California
ORIGIN Mediterranean
U.S.? Yes
FAT (⅓ cup) 19 grams; 2 grams saturated

Cashews

Imported from India and Brazil
ORIGIN: Brazil
U.S.? No
FAT (⅓ cup) 21 grams; 4 grams saturated

Chestnuts

North American chestnut destroyed by blight; now crossbreeds of Asian species
ORIGIN North America, Europe, Asia
U.S.? Yes
FAT (⅓ cup) 0.5 gram; 0 gram saturated

Coconut

Hairy shells 5 or 6 inches across
ORIGIN Tropics
U.S.? Yes
FAT (⅓ cup) 17 grams; 15 grams saturated

Filberts (Hazelnuts)

Sold in shell; squarish nut, hearty flavor
ORIGIN Europe
U.S.? Yes
FAT (⅓ cup) 28 grams; 2 grams saturated

Macadamia Nuts

Soft, round, buttery nut
ORIGIN Australia
U.S.? Yes
FAT (⅓ cup) 33 grams; 5 grams saturated

Peanuts

Technically a legume, not a nut
ORIGIN Brazil
U.S.? Yes
FAT (⅓ cup) 24 grams; 3.5 grams saturated

Pecans

Native to U.S., rich, buttery flavor
ORIGIN Mississippi River Valley, U.S.
U.S.? Yes
FAT (⅓ cup) 24 grams; 2 grams saturated

Pine Nuts

Buttery-tasting seeds from pinecones
ORIGIN North America, Europe, Asia
U.S.? Yes
FAT (⅓ cup) 24 grams; 4 grams saturated

Pistachios

Light green nut
ORIGIN Mediterranean, Asia
U.S.? Yes
FAT (⅓ cup) 20 grams; 2.5 grams saturated

Pumpkin and Squash Seeds

Green, thin, half-inch long; called pepita
ORIGIN Americas
U.S.? Yes
FAT (⅓ cup) 4 grams; 1 gram saturated

Sesame Seeds

Small tan seeds, bland unless roasted
ORIGIN Mediterranean, Asia
U.S.? Yes
FAT (⅓ cup) 24 grams; 3.5 grams saturated

Sunflower Seeds

One flower makes 100 or more seeds
ORIGIN North America
U.S.? Yes
FAT (⅓ cup) 24 grams; 2.5 grams saturated

Walnuts

Black walnuts grow wild in North America
ORIGIN North America, Asia
U.S.? Yes
FAT (⅓ cup) 20 grams; 2 grams saturated

Eat Fresh Produce: Vegetables

Eat your vegetables. We've heard it a thousand times, and for good reason. Or, as Michael Pollan puts it, "Eat food. Not too much. Mostly plants."

The Harvard School of Public Health recommends at least nine servings (4½ cups) of vegetables and fruits a day. (Potatoes don't count!) Go for a variety of types and colors for the mix of nutrients your body needs. Best bets? Dark leafy greens, cooked tomatoes, and anything that's a rich yellow, orange, or red color for their antioxidant value. Variety is the key. Get out of your produce rut and explore eating new types of vegetables.

ARTICHOKES Artichokes—actually the bud of a type of thistle—peak in March through May. Nearly all sold in the United States are from California. Look for large, compact globes with uniform firmness. Artichokes are usually steamed or stuffed. Small artichokes can be eaten whole. Fresh, young artichokes can be eaten raw.

Artichokes contain powerful phytonutrients: cynarin and silymarin. One large globe contains only 25 calories, no fat, 170 milligrams of potassium, along with vitamin C, folate, and magnesium, and has 6 grams of dietary fiber.

ASPARAGUS Asparagus is harvested from March through June, depending on where you are—early asparagus is pencil-thin and the spears thicken as the season progresses. Most people assume that the thinner the spear, the more tender, but usually tenderness has to do with freshness, not thickness. Look for fresh, crisp stalks with compact tips.

Asparagus is versatile; it can be roasted, grilled, steamed, boiled, sauteed, pureed, and eaten raw. It is rich in vitamins A and C, as well as folacin, selenium, potassium, fiber, and thiamine, and is one of the richest sources of rutin, a compound that strengthens capillary walls.

Imported nuts tax the environment. Some must be shipped thousands of miles to your kitchen. But many nuts grow in abundance in North America: almonds, filberts, sunflower seeds, pecans, peanuts, walnuts, and chestnuts. Foragers can also find acorns, hickory nuts, and walnuts.

Don't eat lima beans raw; they contain linamarin, which releases a cyanide compound when the seed coat is opened. It is deactivated once the bean is cooked.

BEANS, FRESH Fresh beans come in two categories: edible-pod beans and shell beans. Green beans (snap or string beans) are the most popular edible-pod bean in the United States. Beans can be cooked whole, cut crosswise, or French-cut (along the length of the bean). The less you cut the bean, the crisper it will be after cooking. Lima beans and edamame (young soy beans) are popular types of shell beans. Both require cooking.

BEETS This root vegetable has two edible parts, the root and its greens. Beets are grown in more than 30 states and provinces, with a peak season of June through October, though they are available year-round. They come in a wide array of shapes, colors, and sizes. Look for firm, smooth roots that are free of splits, cuts, and bruises. For beets without their greens attached, store in the coolest part of the refrigerator for up to one week. The greens perish more quickly and should be eaten as soon as possible. Beets can be baked, steamed, pickled, and used in condiments—they are equally delicious raw. To use the greens, remove them from the roots as soon as possible to prevent wilting and remove the leaves from the thick stems. Beet greens have some of the sweetness of the roots combined with a complex vegetal bitterness. They are great for steaming or sauteing. Beets are an excellent source of folate and a good source of potassium and vitamin C.

Red bell peppers contain 11 times more beta-carotene than green bell peppers.

BELL PEPPERS Bell peppers come in a variety of colors, shapes, sizes, and flavors. Green and purple peppers are very slightly bitter, while red, orange, and yellow peppers are sweeter and fruity. Look for peppers with firm and smooth skin, and without dents or discoloration. The stem should be fresh and green and the pepper should feel heavy for its size. Store unwashed bell peppers in the refrigerator for a week, and wash before using.

BOK CHOY Bok choy, also known as pak choi (which means white vegetable) is a type of cabbage—but it looks like a mix of celery stalks and romaine leaves. It is an excellent source of vitamin C and vitamin A, and a good source of folate and calcium. Select heads with dark green, glossy leaves and bright white stalks. Brown spots on the leaves can indicate poor storage and a loss of flavor. Baby bok choy can be cooked whole; older bok choy can be cut before cooking. Tear the leaves from the stalks, slice the stalks crosswise, and cut the leaves coarsely. Bok choy can be used in salads or can be steamed, braised, sauteed or stir-fried.

BROCCOLI In the United States, the most common type of broccoli available commercially is the Italian green or sprouting variety—recognized by its green stalks topped with domed clusters of green florets. Other varieties

Shopping & Saving

HOW TO KEEP PRODUCE FRESH

The key to keeping produce fresh is to keep it hydrated.

Most produce likes dampness, which is why you see machines or people misting produce at markets. It's best to keep the air in your refrigerator crisper drawer as damp as possible for produce that requires high relative humidity. Some refrigerators do this with a sliding vent—keep it closed for the highest humidity. Keep foods that don't like moisture, such as dried garlic, outside the refrigerator altogether.

These like **high relative humidity** (90%–100%): leafy greens, beans, cucumber, asparagus, broccoli, celery, avocado, berries, green onions, pears.

These like **medium relative humidity** (80%–90%): melons, sweet potatoes, tomatoes, citrus.

These like **low relative humidity** (below 80%): dried garlic, onions, pumpkins, squash.

include the unique-looking Romanesco (a lighter green with pointed, cone-shaped florets); Chinese broccoli (slightly bitter with thick stems, flat leaves, and small florets); and broccoli rabe (also known as rapini, it is bitter with spiked leaves surrounding small stalks of florets).

When selecting broccoli, look for bunches that have rich color, as the more vivid green, purplish, or blue-green florets contain more beta-carotene and vitamin C than yellow or fading ones. Avoid broccoli with open, flowering, or discolored florets and tough or limp stems. Store broccoli unwashed, and wrap the greens in paper towels in the crisper drawer of the refrigerator for several days. Before cooking, trim thick, tough leaves, and rinse well to remove sand and dirt. Broccoli can be eaten raw, or cooked in just about any way—it's an excellent source of the vitamins K, C, and A, as well as folate and fiber.

How to Cook an Artichoke

An artichoke can be an intimidating beast—how does one handle these odd balls of leaves? Once you've mastered the art of preparing them, the only mystery remaining will be how they taste so wonderful.

1. Wash artichokes under cold running water. Pull off any lower petals that are small or discolored.

2. Cut stems close to base. (Use stainless knives to prevent discoloration.)

3. Cut off top quarter and tips of petals, if desired. (Some people like the look of clipped petals, but it really isn't necessary to remove the thorns. They soften with cooking and pose no threat to diners.)

4. Plunge into acidified water to preserve color. (Add 1 tablespoon vinegar or lemon juice per quart of water.)

5. Optional: The trimmed artichoke stems are edible. Cut brown end about ½ inch. Peel fibrous outer layer to reach tender green of stem. Stem may be steamed whole with the artichoke.

Broccoli is a very good source of phosphorus, potassium, magnesium, and the vitamins B_6 and E.

BRUSSELS SPROUTS Although they look just like tiny heads of cabbage (and are in the same family), Brussels sprouts have a sweeter, milder taste. Most Brussels sprouts in the United States are grown in California, with a peak growing season from autumn through early spring. Choose firm, compact sprouts that are bright green in color with tight-fitting leaves. Yellow or wilted leaves indicate lack of freshness or mishandling—and the older the sprouts, the stronger the cabbage flavor will be. Aim to buy sprouts of similar size so they will cook uniformly. Before cooking, trim the ends and use a paring knife to score an X in the stem end; this will help the stem cook more in pace with the leaves.

Brussels sprouts can be boiled, steamed, roasted, stir-fried, or sauteed. Try cutting them into coins or shredding them before cooking to reduce cooking time and for a crisper presentation. Brussels sprouts are an excellent source of vitamin C and a good source of vitamin A, folate, and potassium.

According to the USDA, a diet rich in fruits and vegetables may reduce the risk of stroke and other cardiovascular diseases; certain cancers, such as mouth, stomach, and colon-rectum cancer; kidney stones; type-2 diabetes; and bone loss.

CABBAGE Look for tight, heavy heads of cabbage, avoiding those with discoloring or pest damage. Be wary of precut cabbage, which can quickly lose its vitamin C content. Cabbage can keep up to a week or more in cold storage. Use raw in slaws; for cooking, steam or saute. Cabbage is an excellent source of vitamin C and a good source of vitamin A.

CARROTS There are numerous types of carrots, but the typical ones found in supermarkets are either the ones about 8 inches long, or prepackaged "baby" carrots (which are actually longer carrots that have been mechanically peeled and trimmed). Carrots have a very high natural sugar content, second only to beets among vegetables. Look for carrots with the deepest orange color, which indicates higher levels of beta-carotene; avoid carrots that are crackled, shriveled, soft, or wilted. Eat them raw or roast, boil, steam, glaze, saute, or puree them. Flavors that complement carrots include dill, tarragon, ginger, mint, honey, brown sugar, parsley, lemon, or orange juice. Carrots are an excellent source of vitamin A.

CAULIFLOWER An autumn vegetable, cauliflower is like its relative broccoli while growing, but rather than sprouting green florets, it forms a tight dome of undeveloped white buds. The heavy leaves that cover the plant shield the flower buds from the sun, preventing the chlorophyll (and color) from developing. When buying cauliflower, look for heads that are bright white

SNAPSHOT **HIROMI SHINYA**

“I consider foods containing many enzymes as good food, and I consider foods with few or no enzymes as bad food.”

New York, New York

Professor of Surgery, Albert Einstein College of Medicine

Author, *The Enzyme Factor*

The fresher the vegetables, fruits, and fishes are, the more enzymes they have, explains surgeon and author Hiromi Shinya. To him, flavor means enzymes. “When we eat fresh food,” he says, “it usually tastes good because it is packed with plenty of enzymes.” For that reason, Dr. Shinya suggests increasing the raw food in your diet. “Since enzymes are sensitive to heat, the more you cook something, the more enzymes are lost. Enzymes will break down between 118.4°F and 239°F.”

or cream-colored, firm, and compact, without splotches or browning. Store in the crisper, stem side up to avoid moisture buildup. Eat cauliflower raw, steamed, or sauteed. Or roast the whole head tossed with olive oil, bread crumbs, and Parmesan cheese. Cauliflower is an excellent source of Vitamin C and a good source of folate and fiber.

CELERY ROOT Also called celeriac, celery root is common in French cooking—and although a big, rough, knobby celery root is not very pretty, it has a silky texture with subtle celery and parsley flavors. Peak harvest season is November through April, but roots are available year-round. Select roots that have the smoothest skin for easier peeling; roots larger than a grapefruit will be woody inside. Celery roots should be scrubbed, trimmed, and peeled, with spongy parts thrown away. Celery root can be braised, boiled, roasted, and used in soups, stews, purees, or added to mashed potatoes.

CHARD, SWISS CHARD It's hard to miss these big red or green leaves attached to white, red, or yellow stalks. Chard is available from spring through fall with peak season from June through October. Look for Swiss chard that has crisp stalks and bright leaves. Chard can be kept in the refrigerator for about two days. Chard is similar to beet greens in taste—mildly sweet yet slightly bitter. Tear the leaves from the stem and cook stems first, then leaves. Chard can be used wherever spinach or beet greens are used. Swiss chard is an excellent source of vitamins A and C.

COLLARD GREENS Collard greens are at their peak harvest from January through April—the best are bright and crisp, with leaves intact. Fresh collards should be stored in the crisper drawer of the refrigerator or in a plastic bag with holes in it. Remove thick, tough leaves, and rinse as

As fruits and vegetables age, they give off ethylene gas, which hastens ripening and brings on rotting. Special plastic bags that let you store produce longer use zeolite, a mineral that neutralizes ethylene. The bags are made of polyethylene. (Because of that, never microwave these bags.) There is a plastic-free alternative that works the same way: special disks to put into the crisper drawer also neutralize ethylene gas. It's a technique that has been used by florists and produce distributors for years.

necessary to remove sand and grit. Blanching quickly in simmering water reduces bitterness. Cook in a skillet with small amount of olive oil until just wilted, or steam using the moisture that clings to greens after washing. The traditional Southern way to prepare collards is to simmer them slowly for a long time with a ham hock—resulting in very soft leaves with little bitterness and a vitamin-laden broth best soaked up with corn bread. Collard greens are an excellent source of vitamins A and C and a good source of folate.

Try grilling corn on the cob. Soak corn in husks in cold water for ten minutes. Drain and then grill the husked corn on a rack set five to six inches above glowing coals until husks are charred, about ten minutes. Shuck corn and grill further, until kernels are browned in spots, about ten minutes more.

CORN Americans consume about 25 pounds of corn per person annually. That's a lot—although not that much of it is fresh, whole corn on the cob. When shopping for fresh corn, look for ears with husks that are green and crisp—and pull back the husk to see that the kernels are plump and healthy. Also check that the kernels at the tip are smaller, as large kernels at the end indicate that the corn was picked too late.

Corn should be stored in a cool area—warmth causes the sugar in corn to be converted, resulting in less sweet, more starchy kernels. If you can't cook the corn right away, store it in the refrigerator to retain flavor and vitamin C. Traditionally, corn is boiled in salted water, but you can also grill it.

CUCUMBER The most common cucumber varieties in the American market are Persian and English. Persian cucumbers, the most familiar, are soft with edible seeds and skin that is often waxed to seal in moisture. English cucumbers, also called "burpless" or seedless cucumbers, are longer and thinner with a thinner skin. They are usually wrapped in plastic to seal in moisture. Select firm cucumbers with good color and no bruises or mushy parts. Cucumbers that have a bulge in the middle are usually bloated with watery seeds and will have less

Creative Crudités

Nothing says fresh like crudités—but crudités may seem boring and bland to those accustomed to gooey cheese hors d'oeuvres. To create a stand-out crudité plate, think outside the ranch-dressing box.

Veggie Variety

A twist in vegetable selection can be fun.

- All white (cauliflower, jicama, peeled new potatoes, turnips) for an elegant winter party
- A big bowl with a jumble of whole artichokes for a rustic feel

Or use traditional vegetables in all new ways:

- Cucumber spears instead of coins
- Real baby carrots with stems still attached rather than carrot sticks
- Whole baby squash instead of spears or coins

Or mix it up by adding unexpected vegetables:

- Lightly steamed asparagus
- Sliced fennel
- A few whole artichokes, or stacks of artichoke leaves
- Long slender green beans
- Steamed baby potatoes
- Portabello mushroom slivers
- Jicama spears
- Blanched Brussels sprouts
- Belgian endive leaves

Leek and Goat Cheese Dip

2 tablespoons olive oil
2 medium leeks, white and pale-green parts only, washed well and thinly sliced
1 16-ounce container low-fat Greek yogurt
1 14-ounce log of fresh, creamy goat cheese
1 tablespoon chopped cilantro
1 tablespoon chopped fresh flat-leaf parsley
Salt and pepper

1. In a medium sauteing pan, heat olive oil over medium-low heat. Add leeks and saute until soft and translucent, about 5 minutes.

2. Place yogurt and goat cheese in a medium bowl, and stir until well combined. Add leeks, cilantro, parsley, salt, and pepper. Serve.

flavor. Cucumbers can be refrigerated for up to a week. If you buy or harvest fresh cucumbers that haven't been waxed, wrap them to keep in moisture when stored.

Although cucumbers can be cooked, they are usually eaten raw—in salads, cold soups, hors d'oeuvres, and snacks. They are also used to make raita and tzatziki—yogurt-based cucumber sauces used in Indian and Greek cuisine. Cucumbers are a good source of potassium and fiber with moderate amounts of vitamins A and C, folic acid, phosphorous, and magnesium.

Food irradiation to kill bacteria has been approved in the United States for various foods, including fruit and vegetables. Ask your produce manager to label irradiated produce, since you may want to avoid it.

EGGPLANT The peak growing season for eggplants is July to October. In the United States we most commonly find two varieties of dark purple eggplant in the market: oval and elongated, often called Japanese eggplant. Specialty varieties include Chinese eggplants (light purple and skinny) and rosa biancos (white with violet streaks).

Buy eggplants that have taut, unblemished skin. Supersize eggplants may be tough and bitter. To check for freshness, press in with your finger—the fresher the eggplant, the quicker the skin will bounce back. Eggplants bruise easily. Store them in the refrigerator.

To prepare, wash and remove cap and stem. The skin can be eaten, but in larger varieties the skin is tough and should be peeled before eating. Eggplant is one of the few vegetables whose texture improves with longer cooking. Bake a whole eggplant by piercing the skin with a fork several times, and cooking it at 400°F for about 40 minutes. The resulting soft interior can be pureed or mashed, and the charred skin adds a subtle smokiness. Eggplant can be broiled, sauteed, and stewed: a classic ratatouille.

JICAMA This tuberous root looks like a potato or turnip with tan skin and white flesh. It is eaten raw in Mexico and South America. Its flavor is reminiscent of pear and potato, and it's crisp like a water chestnut. For use in

Healthy for You

CSAs: SHARE THE LOCAL HARVEST

Joining a CSA—community-supported agriculture—is the next best thing to having your own garden. CSAs involve a community of people supporting a local garden or farm either by work or by paying a share of expenses. For this contribution they are entitled to a season's fresh fruits and vegetables (or more, such as milk and honey, depending on the CSA). The CSA can either have an arrangement with a particular farm, or it can lease farmland and hire its own gardener or farmer to work it.

There are probably as many formulas for how to run a CSA as there are CSAs (hundreds around the country). Some CSAs are strict proponents of biodynamic farming—following the basic principles of nature as defined by Rudolf Steiner's biodynamic farming philosophy. These CSAs are farm-centered, meaning that they are part of an established farming philosophy that is often biodynamic and at least organic and sustainable.

Members of a farm's CSA help ensure the farm's economic viability. One farmer who needed a guaranteed local outlet for his produce developed a CSA and managed to keep his struggling farm in business.

Some CSAs are simply loose groups of people who share the work and expenses of an organic garden. The group pools resources to lease or rent land, hires a farmer or gardener (or shares in the gardening), and handles administrative jobs. Members are entitled to a share of the season's harvest, usually 20 weeks of fruits and vegetables.

The great benefit of being a member of a CSA is a season's supply of freshly picked produce, often organic, in all its variety and economy. A CSA also can be a way for people in a community to support family farms in the vicinity. Most CSAs require the member's share of expenses to be paid up front so the grower can buy seeds and other equipment, and thus there is some risk of losing the investment in case of drought or flood. Balance that with the more likely benefit: fresh produce all season long.

Guide to Mushroom Varieties

Mushrooms are available and versatile, and they add flavor and texture to meat-free dishes. They provide important minerals and are one of the few natural sources of vitamin D. Select firm mushrooms with smooth surfaces, dry but not dried out. Refrigerate them up to a week in the packaging they came in. Never store mushrooms in airtight containers—they get slimy. Raw mushrooms don't freeze well, but cooked mushrooms can be frozen for up to one month. To clean mushrooms, brush off any dirt with your fingers or a damp paper towel, rinse briefly under running water, and pat dry. Never soak mushrooms.

White Mushrooms

White mushrooms represent about 90 percent of all mushrooms consumed in the United States. They have a fairly mild taste that intensifies when cooked and blends well with almost anything. They can be cooked or tossed raw in salads.

Crimini Mushrooms (Baby Portabellos)

Similar in appearance to whites, crimini mushrooms have a tan or brown cap and a deeper, earthier flavor. Saute, broil, or cook them almost any way. Their full-bodied taste makes them an excellent addition to beef, wild game, and vegetable dishes.

Portabello Mushrooms

A larger relative of criminis, portabellos have tan or brown caps that measure up to six inches across. They have a meatlike texture and flavor. They can be grilled, broiled, or roasted and served as appetizers, entrees, or side dishes. Their hearty taste and texture make them a flavorful vegetarian alternative—grill and serve them on toasted buns.

Enoki Mushrooms

With tiny, button-shaped caps and long spindly stems, enoki mushrooms are mild and crunchy. Clean by trimming roots at cluster base. Separate stems before serving. Try them raw in salads and sandwiches or use them as an ingredient in soups.

Oyster Mushrooms

Oyster mushrooms can be gray, pale yellow, or even blue, with a velvety texture. They have a very delicate flavor, brought out when you saute them with butter and onions. Try over linguine with sliced steak and red peppers, sprinkled with grated Parmesan cheese.

Maitake Mushrooms

Rippled and fan-shaped, without caps, maitake—also called hen of the woods—have a distinctive aroma and a rich, woodsy taste. Saute lightly in butter or oil. For a richer taste in any recipe calling for mushrooms, use maitakes. They can be a main-dish ingredient or used in side dishes and soups.

Shiitake Mushrooms

Tan to dark brown with broad, umbrella-shaped caps, wide open veils, tan gills, and curved stems that should be removed, shiitakes have a meaty texture and a rich, woodsy flavor when cooked. They add substance and character to stir-fries, pasta, soup, entrees, and side dishes.

salads, remove the peel, including the fibrous flesh directly under the skin. Slice and serve raw, saute, or stir-fry—it stays crisp when cooked. A one-pound jicama produces about three cups chopped or shredded flesh.

Jicama is available year-round but best between November and June. Choose jicama that is free of bruises, cuts, and discoloration. It should feel firm with a dry, not soggy, root. Store whole jicama as you would potatoes or sliced jicama in a refrigerated bowl of water with a squeeze of citrus.

KALE This dynamo of nutrition, part of the cabbage family, is full of disease-fighting attributes, including vitamins A and C. Shop for crisp, tender, bright green leaves. At home, break up the bunch and wash the leaves several times in a sinkful of water, then spread them out on a bath towel. Roll up the towel and gently press to remove excess water. If you are going to use the kale the same day, you can refrigerate it in the rolled-up towel; otherwise, bag it in the crisper drawer.

Kale is versatile: Toss it into salads raw or cook it. You can quickly saute it, but be sure the leaves are thoroughly dry, so that you aren't steaming them.

Try kale chips: Tear kale leaves off stems, toss in olive oil and salt, and roast at 375°F for 15 to 20 minutes until leaves are slightly browned and a little bit crunchy.

KOHLRABI Kohlrabi is a part of the cabbage family and tastes like a mix of broccoli and radish. It may look like a root vegetable, but it grows above the soil line. Kohlrabi is a good source of vitamins and minerals, especially vitamin C. There are two varieties of kohlrabi: purple (sweeter) and green. Select smaller vegetables, no more than two and a half inches in diameter; larger kohlrabi should be peeled before eating. Kohlrabi can be refrigerated for up to a month. Serve the leaves and trimmed bulb raw in salad. You can also steam, saute, and stir-fry kohlrabi. To steam, cook in a covered pot and steam for 10 to 12 minutes. Cook until tender but not mushy.

LEEKS Leeks look like giant green onions. They have a distinctly onion flavor, but they are mild and sweet. A good source of vitamin C, they are best fully cooked. Look for firm and bright white roots, with crisp green leaves. They will refrigerate for at least five days. Leeks often have silt lodged between the layers, so it's important to wash well—slice lengthwise and check for dirt. Most recipes call for the white base only, but leek greens can be used as well.

Leeks are amazing braised or slowly sauteed. They cook into a creamy, melt-in-your mouth texture. If you don't like strong onion flavor, substitute subtle leeks in any recipe calling for onion. They make a great substitute for shallots, too.

MUSTARD GREENS These fierce greens can be tough, bitter, spicy—and wonderful! They come in red or green and are a staple of Southern cooking. They are most commonly braised or slowly cooked, but young tender raw leaves can be a lively addition when added to salads.

Some growers, packers, and distributors artificially color the skins of yellow varieties of sweet potatoes with a red dye. The FDA now deems these sweet potatoes "adulterated"; if you cut them open and find the inside to be yellow, and the outside red, the sweet potatoes are suspect—they have probably been artificially dyed. Report any such sweet potatoes to the produce manager.

OKRA This tall-growing, warm-season, annual vegetable, in the same family as hollyhock and hibiscus, is a staple in Southern cooking. It plays a starring role in gumbo and is also used in soups, pickles, stews, and on its own as a side dish, fried or boiled. Okra is an excellent source of soluble fiber, in the form of gums and pectins, and insoluble fiber. Half a cup provides nearly 10 percent of the recommended levels of vitamin B_6 and folic acid.

Refrigerate okra unwashed—wet pods become slimy—by wrapping it loosely in perforated plastic bags. Okra keeps for only two or three days, but may be frozen for up to a year after blanching whole for two minutes.

PARSNIPS Parsnips look like pale carrots, and they are related to carrots, celery, and parsley. Commonly found in

Healthy for You

WHAT ABOUT THAT WAX?

When you see and feel apples or peppers in the grocery store with a glossy, oily shine, they have probably been waxed. Many fruits, vegetables, and nuts receive a wax coating that may not be so identifiable: eggplants, grapefruit, grapes, or tomatoes, for example. When these waxes are applied on produce already treated with pesticides, the pesticides cannot be washed off.

Federal law requires retailers to display a sign prominently identifying fresh fruits and vegetables that are treated with postharvest wax or resin coating. The sign must read "coated with food-grade animal-based wax, to maintain freshness," or "coated with food-grade vegetable-, petroleum-, beeswax-, and/or shellac-based wax or resin, to maintain freshness," as appropriate. Make sure the stores you shop at display such a sign. And always peel the waxed skin off produce before you eat it or cook with it.

Europe, this root vegetable arrived in North America with the colonists. It has a sweet and nutty flavor and is an excellent source of vitamin C and folate. Parsnips are available year-round, but their peak season is from fall into spring. Larger roots can have a tough, woody core that should be removed. Look for firm roots, and select smaller parsnips, which require less peeling and coring. Avoid limp, pitted, or shriveled roots.

Wash, peel, and trim parsnips as you would carrots. The skins will slip off after steaming, but if you are pureeing the parsnips, leave the skins on. Parsnips are versatile—use them in soups, stews, steamed, roasted, and boiled. They make great baked "fries" and can be boiled and mashed along with potatoes.

Store parsnips unwashed, wrapped in a paper towel inside plastic, in the vegetable crisper for about two weeks.

PEAS: SNOW PEAS AND SNAP PEAS Snow peas and snap peas, eaten pod and all, are excellent sources of vitamin C. Snow peas are flat; snap peas bulge a little. Look for bright green, firm pods; avoid any that are limp or rubbery. Wash them and remove any strings prior to cooking. Snow and snap peas can be boiled, steamed, sauteed, or stir-fried, making sure not to overcook so that they retain their sweet crispness.

Vegetable scraps are filled with flavor and vitamins. Use them for vegetable stock or freeze for future use. Toss leftover salad in a blender with tomatoes or tomato juice and make an instant gazpacho or vegetable juice.

POTATOES Potatoes may be called root vegetables, but they are actually swollen stems. An average five-ounce potato with skin gives 45 percent of the daily requirement of vitamin C, 620 mg potassium (comparable to bananas, spinach, and broccoli), and trace amounts of folate, iron, magnesium, phosphorous, riboflavin, thiamine, and zinc—all for 110 fat-free calories. Skin-on potatoes are an excellent source of fiber—about 2 grams per serving.

One important variable is starch content. High-starch potatoes, like russet varieties, are best for baking, mashing, frying, or pureeing. They cook dry, resulting in fluffy baked potatoes, light mashed and pureed potatoes, and crispy-outside-tender-inside French fries. Low- to medium-starch potatoes, like the red-skinned variety, are somewhat waxy and best for boiling, steaming, braising, and stewing and for recipes where maintaining shape is important, such as potato salad. New potatoes are freshly harvested young potatoes of any variety, and are best used quickly, boiled, steamed, or roasted.

Look for potatoes that are firm, smooth, and fairly clean. Avoid those with wrinkled or wilted skins, soft dark areas, discoloration, cut or bruised surfaces, or greening. Store potatoes in a cool, dark, well-ventilated area. Do not refrigerate or freeze.

PUMPKIN Canned pumpkin is easy, but freshly roasted pumpkin is far better. Skip jack-o'-lantern pumpkins and look for pie, cooking, "sugar," or heirloom varieties of pumpkin. An excellent source of vitamins A and C and a good source of folate, they keep for a month in a cool, dry place or up to three months refrigerated.

To prepare, halve the pumpkin crosswise and scoop out the strings and seeds. (Save and roast the seeds for a snack!) Place halves, hollow side down, in a large baking pan with a little water added. Bake uncovered at 375°F for one and a half to two hours or until fork-tender. Puree cooled pulp in a food processor or blender. To use fresh pumpkin puree in recipes, drain first: Line a strainer with a double layer of cheesecloth or a dish towel and let the pumpkin sit on it for 20-30 minutes.

RADISHES Fresh, crisp radishes have a great crunchy texture and a bright, spicy bite, and provide potassium, vitamin C, folate, and fiber. They are members of the cruciferous vegetable family, so you can eat their greens as well. They are classified as summer radishes—the small vibrant ones, red, pink, purple, white, or red and white, with a flavor ranging from very hot to mild—or winter radishes, such as daikon, which may be white, black, or green. Refrigerate summer radishes in plastic bags for up to a week, winter radishes for up to two weeks.

RUTABAGAS A rutabaga looks like a turnip with yellow-orange flesh and ridges at its neck. They are common ingredients in Scandinavian cooking. They have a delicate sweetness and provide plenty of vitamins A and C. They store well and are available year-round. Look for fresh rutabagas in early autumn, when their flavor peaks. To cook, peel and cut into cubes, then boil for 10 to 15 minutes. You can mash and serve them alone or add to mashed potatoes.

Guide to Salad Greens

What a choice of salad greens we have today, from mild to full-flavored. Select lettuce that feels crisp and fresh, avoiding leaves that are wilting or brown. Lettuce keeps best in plastic bags in the crisper drawer of the refrigerator. Iceberg lettuce lasts two weeks, romaine around ten days, and butterheads and endives around four days. More delicate greens don't even last that long.

Arugula (Rocket)

Arugula has small, flat leaves on long stems and a peppery flavor. Some like it on its own; others balance it with milder lettuces.

Belgian Endive (French Endive)

Endive is characterized by its very pale color and tightly packed, oblong leaves. It is bitter, but not overwhelmingly so.

Butterhead (Boston and Bibb)

Loose, wavy heads, light green leaves, tender texture, and very mild flavor. Boston is the most popular; it looks like a relaxed blooming flower, while Bibb is more cuplike.

Chicory (Curly Endive)

Not to be confused with Belgian or French endive, chicory (or curly endive) is a ragged, curly-leafed lettuce with dark outer leaves and pale, even yellow interior leaves.

Escarole

Another member of the chicory family, this lettuce looks like a curly lettuce but has a distinctive bitter bite. Escarole is popular in Europe in salads or braised.

Iceberg

Once the most popular—and still the least nutritious—of all lettuces, these pale heads look like cabbage but have a softer texture and a mild flavor.

Leaf Lettuces (Green, Oak, Red)

These varieties don't form lettuce heads but have longer leaves joined at the stem.

Mâche (Lamb's Lettuce)

This very delicate salad green is recognizable by its oblong shape, velvety texture, and mild taste. It is generally quite expensive due to its perishability.

Mizuma

A mild Japanese green with long pointy leaves, mizuma is used in salads or mixed with other greens for stir-frys.

Radicchio

This member of the chicory family looks like red cabbage, but has a bitter bite, topped with sweet. Most radicchio is imported from Italy, but specialty growers are starting to supply the North American market.

Romaine

With the popularity of Caesar salad, romaine has become one of the most common lettuces in the market. Its long leaves join at the stem, with darker, flatter (and more nutritious) exterior leaves surrounding crisper, lighter interior ones.

SALSIFY Salsify is a root vegetable with a mild flavor somewhat akin to artichokes or asparagus. It is a good source of fiber, vitamin C, vitamin B_6, riboflavin, and potassium. Find firm, tapered roots with black or white skin; they will keep in the refrigerator for two weeks. Use salsify in soups or stews or boil it until tender and mash.

Ramps, a regional treasure in Appalachia, are wild leeks gathered only in the spring. If you live near deciduous forests from Canada to Tennessee, you might be able to find them, even in markets. Use them raw or cooked in place of scallions or leeks.

SORREL This wild green (also known as a weed) bursts with a bright lemon zing and is used to perk up salads. It is also terrific when cooked—either sauteed with other greens or used on its own in sorrel soup.

SPINACH A superfood beyond compare, spinach is available year-round, great raw and cooked, an excellent source of vitamin A, and a good source of vitamin C and folate. Young leaves are mild and soft in texture, great for salads or quick sautees; older leaves are flavorful and substantial. Sand and dirt love to hide in spinach's many crevices, so rinse several times to remove all grit.

Healthy for You

HOW TO WASH PRODUCE

- Rinse fresh produce under cold, running tap water.
- Do not wash with detergent.

HOMEMADE SPRAY TECHNIQUE

- Put white distilled or apple cider vinegar in one clean spray bottle, 3 percent hydrogen peroxide in another.
- First spray the produce with the vinegar.
- Next spray the produce with the hydrogen peroxide.
- Repeat, alternating sprays, two or three times.
- Now rinse the produce thoroughly under clear running water.

SUNCHOKES (JERUSALEM ARTICHOKES) These knobby nuggets, tubers of a plant related to the sunflower, are also known as Jerusalem artichokes—a misnomer derived from *girasole,* Italian for sunflower, and because they taste like artichoke hearts. An excellent source of iron and thiamine and a good source of potassium, phosphorus, copper, fiber, vitamin C, and niacin, they can be eaten raw or sauteed, braised, roasted, or steamed. They turn brown by oxidation quickly, so toss with lemon juice.

TURNIPS Another great root vegetable, turnips have a strong flavor. Shop for small to medium compact roots with smooth white and purple skin. Cut off the root and greens; boil for 15 to 25 minutes; add to mashed potatoes and other mashed roots, or to soups and stews. Don't discard the greens—an excellent source of vitamin C, they have a peppery flavor when cooked.

WATERCRESS Watercress is one of spring's first tender greens, with crisp curly stems, glossy round leaves, and a wonderfully peppery taste. Look for it in the wild—although avoid it in streams near cattle and sheep pastures—but it's also more and more common in markets. High in vitamins A and C, watercress is lovely raw in salads, sauteed, or in soup.

WINTER SQUASH Butternut, hubbard, acorn—winter squash is great for eating fresh and local in colder climates; an excellent source of vitamins A and C, potassium, and fiber and a good source of folate and thiamine. Look for compact squashes that feel heavy, with thick, clean skin. Squash can be cubed and boiled or, to bring out the flavor, tossed with a little olive oil, salt, and pepper, and roasted at 350°F for 30 to 45 minutes, or until tender. Use butter, maple syrup, and cayenne pepper to add some punch.

Guide to Summer Squash

These tender, warm-season vegetables are harvested throughout frost-free seasons. Summer squash is harvested before the rind hardens. Picked immature, it is thus considerably lower in nutritional value than winter squash. Nutrients concentrate in the peel, so never peel summer squash. It can be grilled, steamed, boiled, sauteed, fried, or stir-fried.

OP = OPEN POLLINATED

Black Zucchini (OP)
Best-known; greenish-black skin, white flesh

Black Beauty Zucchini (OP)
Slender with ridges; dark black-green

Cocozelle Zucchini (OP)
Dark green with light green stripes; long, slender fruit

Vegetable Marrow White Bush Zucchini (OP)
Creamy greenish color; oblong

Aristocrat Zucchini (hybrid)
Popular variety; waxy; medium green

Chefini Zucchini (hybrid)
Glossy; medium dark green

Classic Zucchini (hybrid)
Medium green; compact bush

Elite Zucchini (hybrid)
Medium green; lustrous sheen; extra early

Embassy Zucchini (hybrid)
Medium green; few spines

Gold Rush Golden Zucchini (hybrid)
Deep gold color; superior fruit quality

Early Yellow Summer Crookneck (OP)
Classic; curved neck; warted

President Zucchini (hybrid)
Dark green with light green flecks

Spineless Beauty Zucchini (hybrid)
Medium dark green

Sundance Yellow Crookneck (hybrid)
Early; bright yellow, smooth skin

Early Prolific Yellow Straightneck (OP)
Light cream color; attractive straight fruit

Goldbar (hybrid)
Golden yellow; upright, open plant

White Bush Scallop (OP)
Old favorite; pale green when immature; tender flesh

Peter Pan Scallop (hybrid)
Light green

Scallopini (hybrid)
All-America Selections award winner

Sunburst (hybrid)
Bright yellow; green spot at the squash's blossom end

Butter Blossom (OP)
Selected for its large, firm male blossoms

Gourmet Globe (hybrid)
Globe-shaped; dark green, with light stripes

Sun Drop (hybrid)
Creamy yellow; oval; may be harvested young with blossoms

Eat Fresh Produce: Fruit

The reasons why we should eat at least 4½ cups of fruits and vegetables daily go way beyond the fact that they are fresh and delicious. They also provide an abundance of strength-building and disease-fighting nutrients. To keep this goal from being a struggle, have a variety of fruits on hand, and experiment with new ones.

TRUE TIP To prevent cut apples from becoming brown, dip them into a solution of one part citrus juice and three parts water.

APPLES Select firm, compact apples without bruises or punctures. Shiny skin often indicates crispness, but it also may indicate an added wax coating. These days, groceries offer multiple varieties, and heirloom varieties can be found at farmers' markets in the fall and winter. Keep apples refrigerated to retain crispness. Apples are a great source of fiber and a good source of vitamin C. It's best to eat apples with the skin on, as almost half of the vitamin C content is just underneath it. Eating the skin also increases the insoluble fiber content.

APRICOTS In late spring or early summer, look for fresh apricots: light orange, plump and firm, with a soft fragrance. Place unripe apricots in a paper bag with an apple or banana; the ethylene gas given off by the other fruit will ripen the apricots. Refrigerate ripe apricots.

Try apricots baked in savory rice dishes, diced in grain salads, halved and stuffed with goat cheese, or brushed with honey and grilled for dessert. Apricots rank high in vitamins A and C, provide a good source of potassium, and contain iron, calcium, phosphorus, and fiber.

TRUE TIP Store fruits and vegetables separately. Fruits produce ethylene gas as they ripen, which decreases the storage life of vegetables.

AVOCADOS More than two dozen avocado varieties are grown around the world, but the most common avocado cultivar is the Haas, which is smaller, darker, relatively thick-skinned, and available pretty much year-round in grocery stories. Haas avocados also have creamier flesh and a higher fat content than other varieties.

Avocados are ripe when they yield gently to pressure, but sometimes it's hard to tell the difference between ripe and bruised fruit. It should feel uniformly soft, not just in spots. Don't press too hard to judge, because avocados bruise easily. You can buy one hard and ripen it at room temperature for a few days, then refrigerate.

To use, cut lengthwise around the large central pit, twist the sides apart, and then slice each side lengthwise or scoop out the two halves. Acid will stop browning oxidation—sprinkle lemon or lime juice on top. Avocados should be used raw, and are great plain, in salads and sandwiches, and in dips like guacamole.

It's all right to consider one half cup of 100-percent fruit juice as one fruit serving, but the other servings should be whole food, to get the good dietary fiber from the flesh and skins of fruit and vegetables.

SNAPSHOT **ANDREA KANNAPELL & JULIE BESONEN**

"We're doing what we can in New York City to be organic farmers."

New York, New York

Urban organic gardeners

In New York City's East Village, two neighbors, Andrea Kannapell and Julie Besonen, run a two-apartment windowsill gardening cooperative. Julie, whose apartment faces the sunny side of the street, grows rosemary and tarragon in c14lay pots, up to only ten inches in diameter. Andrea, on the shady side, grows tomatoes, oregano, thyme, spearmint, basil and sage. They trade crops accordingly. Because outdoor space is at a premium, they save their compostable food scraps in the fridge, then take them to the community garden on Seventh Street between Avenues B and C, where the Lower East Side Ecology Center keeps a bin right by the gate. They trade them in for cured compost here and replenish their window pots with it periodically. "We're doing what we can in New York City to be organic farmers," says Julie Besonen. Amazingly enough, that's quite a lot.

Puree ripe avocado in a blender with cold vegetable stock, plain yogurt, lime juice, cilantro, salt, and pepper for a delicious summer soup. About 75 percent of avocado's fat is monounsaturated—the good kind. Avocados are an excellent source of vitamins A, C, and E and have about 60 percent more potassium than bananas—as well as one of the highest fiber contents of all fruit.

Cooking & Eating

MEET THE FRUIT DESSERT FAMILY

BETTY
A baked pudding consisting of layers of fruit (usually apples) baked between layers of buttered bread crumbs—related to the French apple charlotte.

BUCKLE
A rich cake with fruit added to the batter—often blueberries—and finished with a streusel topping. It is similar to a coffee cake.

CLAFOUTI
This French cake is usually made with cherries and consists simply of a rich batter poured into a single layer of cherries and baked. Traditionally, the cherry pits are left in to intensify the flavor.

COBBLER
A deep-dish fruit dessert for which biscuit dough is dropped into the fruit before baking—the dessert world's version of chicken and dumplings.

CRISP/CRUMBLE
Easiest of all baked fruit desserts, crisps or crumbles are deep-dish fruit desserts topped with a crumbly pastry mixture, which might consist of flour, nuts, bread crumbs, cookie or graham cracker crumbs, or even breakfast cereal.

GRUNT
A spoon pie with biscuit dough on top, steamed, not baked

PANDOWDY
This dish has fruit on the bottom and a rolled crust on top, which is broken and slightly submerged during baking to allow the juices to bubble through to the top.

SLUMP
Popular in colonial America, a slump is basically a cobbler of fruit with a biscuit or crumb topping, usually cooked on top of the stove.

BANANAS Bananas are one of the most popular fruits in the world, even though this tropical treat isn't local for anyone living in a temperate climate. Granted, they do find their place in many a menu: in peanut butter sandwiches, puddings, baked goods, and pancakes. Sauteed and caramelized, they are delicious with yogurt. Overripe bananas can be peeled and frozen, for later use in baking or smoothies. Bananas are an excellent source of vitamin B_6, fiber, potassium, and vitamin C.

BERRIES In general, buy berries that are plump, symmetrical, and have rich color. For best results, store them in the refrigerator in their original container, and don't wash them until it's time to use them. Gently rinse berries under cool water. Allow them to come to room temperature for the best flavor. Berries are a good to excellent source of vitamin C, and they have excellent antioxidant properties. Each type of berry has something special to offer.

Blackberries range in color from deep blue to purple to black, and are often two-toned. They are very fragile and should be kept dry and refrigerated.

Blueberries are one of the highest-ranking fruits in antioxidant activity. They should have a soft, hazy white coating, which is called "bloom"—it's a natural part of the berries' defense mechanism.

Fresh cranberries should be shiny, deep red, and hard. Those that are soft are overripe and shouldn't be eaten. Frozen cranberries that have been thawed, though, will have a soft texture.

Currants and gooseberries come from the same family—they look like miniature bunches of grapes and come in a variety of colors. These berries are common in jelly and juices, but they are also good in pies and sauces.

Buy strawberries that are clean, plump, and dry with fresh, unwilted caps. Avoid strawberries with seedy tips or white shoulders—those are signs that they were picked too early and will not be very sweet.

Raspberries are extremely fragile. They should be stored dry in your refrigerator, where they will keep only for a few days. Eat them soon after purchase—which shouldn't be hard.

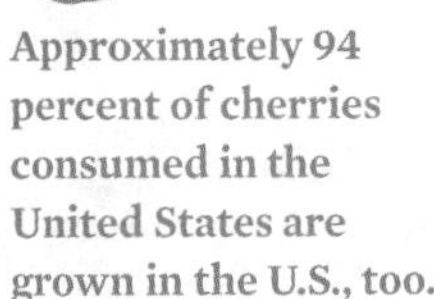

Approximately 94 percent of cherries consumed in the United States are grown in the U.S., too.

CHERRIES Bing cherries are large, deep red, juicy, and sweet. Montmorency cherries are lighter red and tart. Rainier cherries are large and yellow with a red blush, delicately flavored with high sugar levels.

Cherries should be refrigerated immediately after purchase and not left in the sun or warm areas, as they soften quickly. Among fruits, they have comparatively high levels of disease-fighting antioxidants. They also contain important nutrients such as beta-carotene, folate, iron, magnesium, potassium, and vitamin C, plus fiber.

CLEMENTINES This mostly seedless variety of mandarin orange is thin-skinned and sweet—and will keep for three weeks to a month in the refrigerator. Pick ones that feel heavy and compact. They are an excellent source of vitamin C and a good source of fiber and folate.

FIGS Fresh figs have a tender skin, with flesh that ranges from pale yellow to deep rose or purple. They are juicy, crunchy with seeds, and have a sweet and aromatic flavor when ripe—although gummy with latex when unripe. Figs need to ripen fully on the tree and are highly perishable. They will last several days when refrigerated, but should be eaten soon after harvesting. A fresh fig can be peeled and eaten as is or quartered and scooped. Some people eat figs skin and all.

Figs go into cookie bars, pies, puddings, cakes, bread, baked goods, jams, marmalades, and fig paste. Try eating figs with morning cereal, grain dishes, stuffed with goat cheese and pistachios, or poached in wine and served with Greek yogurt. Figs are an excellent source of fiber and have the highest overall mineral content of all common fruits, especially potassium, calcium, and iron.

GRAPEFRUIT Varying in color from light yellow to warm red, the best grapefruits are firm and heavy. Grapefruits can be stored out for seven to ten days, or refrigerated for several weeks. Cut a grapefruit in half and eat it raw or top with a little honey and broil till lightly browned. Add grapefruit sections to salads, toss with avocado and lemon juice, or use in place of any citrus. Grapefruits are an excellent source of vitamin C and fiber and a good source of folate.

Fun, Kids, Pleasure

PEELS AND SKINS = LOVELY LEFTOVERS

- Grate the outer layer of oranges, lemons, or limes to make zest for marinades, baking, and flavored vinegars and oils. You can also freeze zest if you wrap it well.
- Strips of citrus peel are good in cocktails, sparkling water, and tap water—or to make into candied citrus peels.
- Infuse honey, olive oil, or vinegar with citrus peels.
- Rub juiced lemon or lime halves on greasy pans, splattered stovetops, stinky sinks, counters, or cutting boards to clean and refresh.
- For a light skin tonic, rub orange or grapefruit peels on your face (watch out for your eyes!) and then gently rinse with warm water.
- Rub the fleshy part of an avocado peel on your face for a luscious moisturizer.
- Potato peelings are a great puffiness reducer: Press the moist side of the fresh peels to the skin around your eyes for a relaxing 15 minutes.

GRAPES Look for firm, full grapes of whatever variety you prefer. If you are buying imported grapes, buy organic—domestic grapes have a significantly lower pesticide load. Grapes are great for quick and healthy snacks and a sweet accent in salads.

For an unusual preparation, toss grape clusters with olive oil, salt, and pepper and roast on a baking sheet at 450°F for 15 minutes. The skins will be slightly crisp and the centers soft.

Also use in pilafs or salads, or mix with yogurt. Grapes are an excellent source of vitamin C, and purple grapes have an impressive amount of antioxidants.

KEY LIMES Unlike the more common Persian limes, Key limes are smaller—about the size of a golf ball—with a thin, greenish-yellow skin. The flesh inside shares the same hue. They are juicier and have a higher acidity than Persian limes, with that distinctive aroma and tangy flavor for which they are prized.

Cooking & Eating

TOMATO: A FRUIT OR A VEGETABLE?

Botanically speaking, a tomato is a fruit. Like other fruits, tomatoes develop from the ovary in the base of the flower, and contain the seed of the plant.

But in 1893, the U.S. Supreme Court, resolving a dispute over a new vegetable tariff act, ruled this fruit a vegetable. Essentially, since tomatoes were eaten with dinner rather than at dessert time, they were legally determined to be considered a vegetable (and hence taxable!).

Whether you call it a fruit or vegetable, look for heirloom varieties of tomato—these offer more taste, texture, color, and character than typical supermarket varieties. Store tomatoes at room temperature: Refrigerated tomatoes lose their flavor.

KIWIFRUIT Look for fuzzy egg-sized fruits that yield to slight pressure but don't have bruises or soft spots. Kiwifruits are ready to eat when soft. They can be stored at room temperature to ripen and, once ripe, can keep in the refrigerator for several weeks. Surprisingly, even the skin is edible—although rather fuzzy.

Kiwifruit is rich in the protein-dissolving enzyme actinidin, akin to the enzymes found in fresh pineapple, papaya, and figs, which makes it great for your digestive system and for tenderizing meat—but not great for adding to Jell-O, since it prevents the gelatin from setting!

Eat kiwifruit in salads, in salsas, and with meat. It has a high level of dietary fiber and is also an excellent source of vitamin C, plus potassium and vitamins A and E.

KUMQUATS This diminutive member of the citrus family is about one and a half inches long and has a uniquely sweet and tart flavor. Look for thin-skinned kumquats; leaves still attached indicate the freshest fruit. Kumquats can be eaten raw and whole—the skin is the sweetest part, and if you gently roll the fruit between your fingers you will release the essential oils in the rind for the best flavor. Kumquats can also be added to desserts, salads, jellies, jams, marmalade, poached, or put on kabobs and grilled with other fruit, poultry, or meat. Kumquats are a good source of vitamins A and C.

LYCHEES You can find these strawberry-red, rose, or pinkish fruits sold fresh in Asian markets and increasingly in regular supermarkets. Oval, heart-shaped, or nearly round with a thin, leathery, rough or bumpy skin, they are about an inch or an inch and a half long. The flesh ranges from translucent white to gray or pink, somewhat like a grape. They have a distinctively sweet, perfumy flavor.

To peel a lychee, cut off the stem or make a small hole in the fruit. Squeeze the flesh and seed right out.

Lychees are eaten raw and are used in desserts and to garnish savory dishes. They are an excellent source of vitamin C and also provide copper and potassium.

MANGOES Most mangoes range from three to eight inches long and are usually kidney-shaped or ovate. They have a leathery skin, smooth and waxy, that changes to pale green or yellow with red when ripe. Look for smooth-skinned fruit without bruises and allow these fruits to ripen outside the refrigerator.

The flesh of a mango is fibrous, but fragrant, creamy, and very sweet, with notes of flowers and peach. The large flat seed in the middle and the fibrous nature of

---

Preserved Lemons

A staple of Moroccan and Middle Eastern cuisine, preserved lemons add a vibrant, salty zing to just about any type of dish you can think of. They are amazing with poultry, whole grain salads, steamed vegetables, fish, olives, and in relishes.

YOU'LL NEED:
Clean jars and lids
Organic, unwaxed, scrubbed lemons
Additive-free kosher salt

1. Work on the lemons over a bowl or cutting board that will catch the juice. Cut each lemon in quarters lengthwise, but leave the quarters attached at one end so that the lemon remains in one piece.

2. Pour a few tablespoons of salt in the bottom of a jar. Place the split lemons into the jar and pack them with salt, pressing them into the jar, layering them, and topping it all off with more salt.

3. Pour any extra juice into the jar and cover tightly.

4. Leave the jar at room temperature for three days. The lemons should be submerged in juice by then; if not, add more juice.

5. Let the lemons pickle for three weeks. They do not require refrigeration, but many store them in the fridge anyway. They will keep for up to one year. Serve preserved lemons whole, sliced, or diced.

the fruit can make working with mangoes a challenge. Cut two lengthwise lobes off each side parallel to the flat side of the seed, scoop the flesh out from the skin, and then trim as much as you can from the pit.

Eat mangoes plain; use them in smoothies or Indian lassis, or yogurt drinks; or cube them for fruit salad, kabobs, and salsas. Mangoes are an excellent source of vitamins C and A and a good source of fiber. They contain more than 20 different vitamins and minerals.

MEYER LEMONS Meyer lemons are probably a hybrid between a regular lemon and a mandarin orange, accounting for their roundness and their deep yellow-with-slight-orange tint when ripe. They are sweeter, with a distinctive honey taste, and less acidic than supermarket lemons—and thus used in many specialty dishes.

ORANGES What an array of orange varieties we have to choose from. Valencias are in season from February through October, with peak harvest from May to July. They are thin-skinned, sweet, juicy, with some seeds, and excellent for juicing and eating. Blood oranges are streaked and have ruby-red juice. Navel oranges have a second orange at the base of the original fruit; their season lasts from November through May.

Oranges can be stored out or refrigerated for a longer life. They are excellent sources of vitamin C and fiber and good sources of folate.

PAPAYAS There are two types of papayas available in the United States: Hawaiian and Mexican. Hawaiian varieties are pear-shaped and turn from green to yellow when ripe. The flesh is bright orange or pink, dense, and sweet, with a pleasant floral muskiness. Mexican papayas are much larger and can grow to an impressive 15 inches. The flesh is usually dark pink and the flavor less intense than

Slice fruit in small chunks and freeze for smoothies—this works for any fruit, even bananas, oranges, and melons. Later, in a blender, mix the frozen fruit with milk, soy milk, yogurt, kefir, juice, or any combination of the above, and blend until smooth.

the Hawaiian papaya. Look for plump and compact fruit without bruises. If it's hard and greenish, it's not ripe yet. Store it on the counter until it turns yellow and soft and then refrigerate it. Eat within a week.

Papaya contains a protein-dissolving enzyme, papain, which helps digestion and is used to tenderize meat. Papayas are rich in carotenes, vitamin C, flavonoids, folate, pantothenic acid, potassium, magnesium, and fiber.

PEACHES AND NECTARINES Peaches and nectarines are very similar in appearance, flavor, and harvest time. Peaches are classified into three basic categories: clingstone, freestone, and semi-freestone. It all depends on how easily the ripe fruit separates from the pit.

The first to be harvested are clingstone, which ripen from May through August. The flesh is yellow, with bright red touches close to the stone. They are juicier and sweeter than other types, more often found at farms and orchards than the supermarket, and used almost exclusively for canning. The freestone peach harvest begins in late May and continues to October. These are the "eating" peaches that are most commonly found in stores. They tend to be larger, less juicy, and less tender than clingstones. The semi-freestone is a new hybrid, a mix of clingstone and freestone that offers the best of both.

When shopping, look for peaches that are firm but yield with gentle pressure. Don't buy green peaches, as those won't fully ripen. Look for a well-defined cleft and a nice fragrance. Store peaches or nectarines in a cool

We enjoy the comfort and plenty which this highly organized production and distribution system has brought us, but don't we sometimes feel ... that we are in danger of losing all contact with the origins of life and the nature which nourishes it all? **–EUELL GIBBONS, *STALKING THE WILD ASPARAGUS***

place or in the refrigerator for three to five days. They taste best at room temperature. They are a good source of potassium and vitamins A and C.

PEARS Every pear variety has its personality: Anjou pears are mild and firm; Bartletts are the juiciest raw but lose their shape quickly when cooked; Bosc pears are crisp and grainy when raw and hold their shape when cooked; Comice pears are great raw with a fragrant flavor and less grainy texture. Some like pears hard, some like them soft and juicy. Store them on the counter to ripen; refrigerate once they are ripe, when they gently yield to the touch. Use pears in tarts, crisps, cakes, and applesauce, and as a sweet accompaniment to savory dishes. Pears are a good source of vitamin C and fiber.

PERSIMMONS Two varieties of persimmon are grown commercially: Fuyu and Hachiya. Both ripen to a sweet, slippery, floral-scented, and succulent fruit. Look for Hachiyas that are deep orange with no green or yellow, except at the stem. When ripe, they should feel very squishy. Keep them refrigerated and use them within a few days. To expedite ripening, Hachiya persimmons can be kept at room temperature for a week or more.

For Fuyu persimmons, find ones that are yellow-orange and firm. Fuyus will stay firm for two or three weeks at room temperature; when they eventually soften, they have reached their peak sweetness.

Fuyus can be eaten right away, but an unripe Hachiya persimmon is shockingly astringent. Persimmons are used in puddings, baked goods, cheesecakes, jams, and chutneys—and are an excellent source of vitamin C.

PLUMS Most of the plums sold in the United States are known as Japanese plums—round in shape and in a range of colors: red, black, green, or purple. European plums are also available—smaller, oval or teardrop-shaped with purple skin, these are the plums that are dried into prunes. To determine the ripeness of a plum, apply gentle pressure to see if it's beginning to soften. If not yet soft, let the fruit sit for a day or two at room temperature. Ripe plums can be stored in the refrigerator.

Plums are an excellent source of vitamins A and C, calcium, magnesium, iron, potassium, and fiber.

PLUMCOTS, APRIUMS, AND PLUOTS These fairly recent hybrids are mixes of plum and apricot parentage. A plumcot is a cross between an apricot and plum. An aprium is a cross between a plumcot and an apricot and, like an apricot, is slightly fuzzy. A pluot is a cross between a plumcot and a plum. Pluots and apriums are known for their sweetness, as the sugar content of these fruits is greater than that of their parents. Harvest season extends from May to September. When selecting, look for fruit that is plump and firm, avoiding those that are green, blemished, or have broken skin. They can be ripened at room temperature and refrigerated once ripe.

POMEGRANATES Ignore the leathery, wrinkled skin and look for pomegranates that feel compact and plump.

Healthy for You

FRUIT JUICE ALERT

When buying ready-made fruit juice, watch out for beverages named "juice drinks," "cocktails," "fruit punches," and "fruit nectars." They can contain 10 percent or even less juice along with a full range of sweeteners, including high-fructose corn syrup, plus artificial flavors and colors. Read labels carefully to get all juice.

Eat seeds plain, or use them in salads, warm rice pilafs, cool grain salads, relishes, desserts, jams, and syrup.

To remove pomegranate seeds, cut off the crown and then cut the fruit into several sections. Submerge each section in a bowl of cool water and roll the seeds out with your fingers, then strain in a colander.

Pomegranates contain calcium, potassium, and iron, plus a good array of phytonutrients.

QUINCES Quinces look like squat, bumpy yellow pears. The main variety available is the pineapple quince. They can be stored in the refrigerator for a few weeks. An incredibly fragrant fruit, quinces are too astringent, hard, and tart to eat raw. Once cooked, however, the flesh softens, becomes a beautiful ruby purple, and has a perfumed, sweet, yet still tart taste.

Quinces can be peeled and roasted, baked, or poached, and they can be added to favorite recipes whenever a fragrant sweet and tart burst is called for. Most often used for jams, jellies, puddings, and sauces, quinces provide vitamin C, fiber, and riboflavin.

TANGERINES Tangerines are like small oranges, but often sweeter. Look for compact fruits free of bruises and store at room temperature, or longer in the refrigerator. Tangerines are a great snack, delicious in salads, yogurt, or ice cream. They are an excellent source of vitamin C and a good source of fiber and folate.

Fruit a little tired? Puree berries that have passed their prime with lemon juice and honey (and ginger if you like) and freeze into ice cubes to pop into a glass of punch or sparkling water.

I remember how excited we were when the first peaches were ripe because we knew peach cobbler would soon be on the table. We felt the same way when we spied blackberries along the hedgerows, looking forward to the pie Mother would bake. –EDNA LEWIS, *IN PURSUIT OF FLAVOR*

Cooking with Fresh Herbs

Herbs are plants whose leaves are rich in aromatic essential oils, which impart flavor to foods both cold and cooked. Here are some of the tastiest and most widely available herbs, plus a few flavorful seeds and roots. Whenever possible, use them fresh. Next best, dry them yourself. Fresh herbs taste the most vibrant, but they have a high water content. Use more than the dried herb in a recipe.

TRUE TIP

Generally, 1 tablespoon of fresh herbs is equal to about 1 teaspoon of crumbled dried herbs, or 1/4 teaspoon powdered, dried herbs.

ANGELICA Delicate and sweet, somewhat like celery, it is sometimes called wild celery. Angelica stems are often candied and eaten as is or used in cakes and desserts.

ANISE Anise is an herb that is aromatic and sweet, and its seeds are renowned for their licorice-like flavor. Aniseed is used in a wide variety of cuisines and confectioneries, and has long been a popular flavoring for liquors in many countries around the world: Bulgarian *mastika*; the French spirits absinthe, anisette, and *pastis*; Greek ouzo; Arabic arrack; German *Jägermeister*; Turkish raki; Italian *sambuca;* and Colombian *aguardiente.*

BASIL Basil is one of the most popular herbs in the United States and comes in two general varieties: purple and green. Purple basil tends to have smaller leaves and is slightly less sweet than green basil; both share a peppery, minty flavor with a touch of sweetness. The flavor of fresh basil is incomparable—the essence of pesto—and dried basil has quite a different character.

BEE BALM Also known as wild bergamot (but not related to the bergamot citrus), bee balm tastes like oregano and mint, with a little citrus. The leaves are reminiscent of the taste of Earl Grey tea, which is actually flavored with bergamot fruit.

Cooking & Eating

HERBES EN FRANÇAIS!

BOUQUET GARNI: a bunch of fresh herbs, tied with string, used in dishes that are cooked for a long time; the bundle generally contains parsley, bay leaf, and thyme.

FINES HERBES: an herbal combination minced and added as a garnish after cooking; generally contains fresh chervil, parsley, tarragon, thyme, and chives.

BEURRE MAÎTRE D'HÔTEL: another name for compound butter: softened butter creamed together with a dash of olive oil and a mix of chopped fresh herbs, then formed into a log, chilled, and used on meat, fish, vegetables, etc. Compound butter can be frozen and is another good way to store fresh herbs.

BORAGE Young borage leaves can be chopped and eaten raw and have a flavor reminiscent of cucumber. They can be cooked like spinach and also used in soups, stews, and as a garnish. Borage fritters are made by frying battered leaves and sprinkling with sugar.

In general, cooking weakens the flavor of herbs, so add fresh herbs to soups or stews in the last 30 minutes. For chilled foods such as dips, dressings, and marinades, add fresh herbs several hours before serving or overnight to maximize their flavors.

CHERVIL One of the herbs in the fines herbes of French cuisine (see above), chervil is like a delicate mix of anise and parsley. Like both of them, the plant is a member of the carrot family, and the young leaves, which smell like anise, are often used in herb vinegars.

CHIVES Related to onions and other bulb vegetables, chives look like hollow stems of grass and have a fresh, light onion flavor. They are perfect when you want a delicate onion flavor that won't overpower a dish. Delicious on eggs, they often garnish baked potatoes with sour cream.

CILANTRO This herb is also known as coriander leaf, Chinese parsley, *koyendoro,* Mexican parsley, *pak chee, yuen-sai,* green coriander, coriander green, and *dhania*—you can see how many cultures have taken it to be their own. Some people think cilantro is like catnip for humans, while others can't stand the flavor of it. It has a bright, green citrus flavor with a subtle edge—detractors say it tastes soapy. Fresh cilantro can go into salads, salsas, and as a garnish on many dishes, savory and sweet.

The seeds of the cilantro plant go by the name of coriander, and are often used whole or powdered as a seasoning in pickling and making sausage.

DILL Dill has a clean and grassy taste. It is used extensively in Scandinavian and Eastern European cuisine and often paired with fish. It's used generously in a number of international cuisines, and is half the fun of dill pickles. Dill should be used lightly as the flavor has a tendency to intensify. Besides pickles and fish, dill works well with dairy-based dips and sauces and with eggs.

FENNEL All parts of the fennel plant are edible—roots, stalks, leaves, and dried seeds. In some uses it is as much a vegetable as an herb. Every part has a subtle licorice-like flavor, which is more delicate than anise. Fennel is often used in sauces for fish and to season pork roasts and sausages.

TRUE TIP

Leftover herbs can be used to make herb vinegar; stems can go in soup stock. Dried herbs lose their potency over the course of a year, so freshen your supply regularly.

GARLIC Garlic is the bulb of a plant belonging to the lily family—the same family that brings us onions, chives, leeks, and scallions. The bulb, or head, is a cluster of segments referred to as cloves. The cloves should be tightly packed—loose cloves, wrinkled skin, and brown color suggest that the bulb is deteriorating. There are many garlic varieties, from small Southeast Asian varieties to elephant garlic, which can weigh over a pound and is less intense than regular garlic. To make roasted garlic, cut ½ inch off the top of the head, drizzle with olive oil, wrap in aluminum foil, and bake at 400°F for 30 minutes.

Experiment with soaking dried herbs for ten minutes or so before adding to a dish. Soak in water that has just boiled or the hot liquid used for cooking. Heat releases the flavor of the herb.

GINGER There's nothing like the sweet, spicy taste of fresh ginger. Gingerroot is essential to Asian and Indian cuisine, where it is used in chutneys, pickles, and curry pastes. Ginger works in marinades, salad dressings, and soups—as well as in sweet dishes like gingerbread, ginger snaps, and even ginger ale. You'll find pickled ginger accompanying your sushi, and candied ginger as a special confection in a number of desserts. You can leave ginger root in the freezer and grate it, frozen, as needed.

HORSERADISH Horseradish root has a hot, biting flavor that is most potent when raw—as soon as it is cooked, it loses its pungency. Fresh horseradish can be grated after it has been trimmed and scrubbed to remove any soil; discard the woody core, which lacks flavor and is hard to grate. Store the whole root in the refrigerator crisper drawer for up to several weeks. Grated horseradish can also be frozen.

Lemon Verbena Syrup

Lemon verbena's strong floral fragrance makes a delightful syrup to put in tea, sparkling water, savory salad dressings, fruit salad, or on top of pancakes or ice cream—anywhere a sweet and citrusy splash is welcome.

½ cup unrefined sugar
½ cup water
1 cup lemon verbena leaves

1. Mix unrefined sugar and water in a small saucepan, heat to a simmer, and then cool.

2. Place fresh lemon verbena leaves and cooled syrup in a blender and puree on high for 2 minutes.

3. Refrigerate overnight, then strain through a fine strainer or sieve. Store in the refrigerator.

HYSSOP Hyssop has a tangy mint flavor that gives a unique spin to salads, soups, and meat dishes. It is also used often with fruit, and traditionally added to cranberries, cooked peaches, pies, ice cream, and drinks.

LAVENDER Lavender is a member of the mint family, and its flavor is sweet and floral, with a hint of citrus. It is used in hearty game and meat dishes—a great substitute for rosemary—and should be used sparingly or in combination with other herbs to tame its floral power. It is one of the herbs found in the Moroccan blend called *ras el hanout.* Fresh lavender blossoms make a lovely garnish.

LEMON BALM Lemon balm is fragrant with the aroma of lemons. It is sweet and delicate, and thus can be used generously. It complements meat and poultry, but is just as delicious added to salads, fruit drinks, tea, ice cream, jams, and fruit. Because of its delicate flavor, lemon balm should be added at the end of cooking.

LEMON THYME Of the 50 forms of thyme, only three are grown for culinary use, and lemon thyme is one of them.

Many fresh herbs can be dried for later use as well. For more on dried seasonings, a great option for winter months, see pages 256-61.

Cooking & Eating

STORING HERBS

Herbs begin to lose their potency after picking, so try to use them quickly. Refrigerate them in a perforated plastic bag. Before use, wash them gently under cool, but not cold, water and pat them dry between dish towels.

Drying is the classic way to store herbs, but you can also freeze fresh herbs. Wash them gently, dry them, and remove leaves from the stems. Freeze them whole or chopped, packing them into airtight containers.

Lemon thyme's essence is so strong it can actually be used in place of lemon juice or zest. It is great for citrus notes in a marinade or dressing, and works equally with fruit desserts, in jams, and even in custards.

LEMON VERBENA Another of the lemony herbs, lemon verbena has a very pronounced lemon flavor and should be used more sparingly than lemon balm and lemon thyme. It is especially great finely minced and used in fish or chicken dishes, with fruit, and in drinks.

The more finely you chop fresh herbs, the more oils and flavor you release.

LOVAGE Lovage has a distinct celery flavor and should be used sparingly in soups, stews, casseroles, omelets, and salads. The leaves and stalks can also be cooked on their own as a vegetable. Stems can be candied like angelica.

MARJORAM Marjoram is a versatile herb, good mixed with other herbs, and it goes nicely with meats, poultry, and stews. In Mexico, marjoram, thyme, and oregano are mixed to create the earthy and pungent *hierbas de olor,* the Mexican version of the French bouquet garni.

MINT In the United States, we most commonly use peppermint and spearmint; other types include ginger, apple, and curly mint. Mint is a common ingredient in Thai food, Middle Eastern dishes, and in traditional mint tea from North Africa. Mint is delicious paired with salty flavors like feta cheese and is a great match with peas, lamb, chocolate, and fruit.

OREGANO Oregano is slightly sweet and spicy, warm, and a bit bitter. Dried oregano has a much stronger flavor than fresh. Greek oregano, the one popularly found on pizza, is usually milder than Mexican oregano. Oregano is a staple in Italian, Greek, and Spanish cuisine and pairs beautifully with Mediterranean flavors.

PARSLEY The two most famous types of parsley are flat-leafed and curly. Flat, or Italian, parsley has a stronger flavor, with more of a subtle spicy edge, whereas the curly variety is pretty, with a milder flavor. Pasta and egg dishes taste great with parsley, and it is often used to flavor soups and stews. Parsley is a palate cleanser and digestive aid—not just a pretty garnish.

PURSLANE Many gardens sprout purslane as a common weed. Come to know it, and you will find it a lovely green addition to summer meals. Purslane's leaves and stems can be eaten raw and fresh in salads—its lovely clean, acidic flavor makes it a great salad green and makes it pair well with other herbs. It can be cooked as a green or used in soups, broths, salads, and sauces.

Put chopped fresh herbs in an ice cube tray, covered with a bit of water. Pop frozen cubes out and place in an airtight container for whenever a dash of fresh taste is desired.

ROSEMARY Rosemary's pinelike fragrance and hearty flavor make it a perfect match for robust savory dishes, but it's great used lightly in sweet dishes as well. (Think rosemary shortbread cookies, for example.) The herb works especially well with potatoes, bread, pork chops, poultry, and grilled fish.

SAGE The taste of sage runs from mild to peppery, sometimes with a touch of mint—it is one of the main flavors in Thanksgiving turkey stuffing. Because of its strong and distinct flavor, sage pairs particularly well with richer foods, such as sausage, baked chicken, cream-based sauces, and meats. Sage is hearty enough to be added at the beginning of cooking.

SAVORY There are two types of savory: winter and summer. Savory is peppery, and winter savory is a bit stronger than summer savory. This herb has a long tradition in European cuisines as a staple flavoring for beans, meat, and poultry.

TARRAGON Also known as French tarragon, this herb has long, tapered leaves and offers a sweet and subtle anise flavor. It is often used with foods that are delicate in flavor, such as chicken and eggs. A very popular herb in France, tarragon has the starring role in classic béarnaise sauce. Tarragon does not stay fresh for long, which is why it is often added to herb vinegars as a way to extend its life.

THYME Tiny-leaved thyme is strong in flavor, spicy and woody, and pairs well with other herbs such as basil, sage, and lavender, as evidenced by its use in bouquet garni to flavor broths, soups, and stews. Strip the leaves off the woody stems before using the fresh herb.

SNAPSHOT **DEBORAH LEE**

"Why spend all this time getting rid of weeds, when they are the easiest thing to grow?"

Quincy, Illinois

Herbalist and nutritionist

Author, *Exploring Nature's Uncultivated Garden*

Deborah Lee grew up hiking and fishing along the Mississippi River with her grandfather and father. They taught her to identify plants, but it wasn't until many years later, in her own organic garden, that she made foraging part of her life. "There I was, hoeing and mulching, babying along my vegetables, getting rid of the weeds, and I thought, something is wrong here. Why don't I study these weeds? Could they be useful? I wasn't spraying any chemicals, and the weeds looked so happy and vibrant. God put them right in my garden, and maybe I should pay attention." After nine years of eating wild food every day, Lee has discovered that she has an intuition about the nutritional and medicinal qualities of wild plants, and she has also learned that many of her hunches match the ancient teachings of Native Americans.

Edible Flowers

The culinary use of flowers dates back thousands of years to the Chinese, Greeks, and Romans, and many cultures use flowers in their traditional cooking—think of squash blossoms in Italian food and rose petals in Indian food. Preparing dishes with flowers can be a lovely way to add color, flavor, and delight to any meal!

ALLIUM All blossoms from the allium family (leeks, chives, garlic, garlic chives) are edible and flavorful. Flavors run the gamut from delicate leek to robust garlic. Every part of these plants is edible.

ANGELICA Depending on the variety, angelica flowers range from pale lavender-blue to deep rose, and they have a licorice-like flavor.

Healthy for You

EATING FLOWERS SAFELY

- Eat flowers you know to be consumable–if you are uncertain, consult a reference book on edible flowers and plants. When in doubt, don't eat them.
- Eat flowers you have grown yourself, or you know to be safe because you know how they were grown. Flowers from the florist or nursery may have been treated with chemicals and should not be served as food.
- Do not eat flowers picked along the roadside or in public parks. Both may have been treated with pesticides or herbicides, and roadside flowers may be polluted by car exhaust fumes.
- Remove the pistils and stamens and just eat the petals.
- If you suffer from allergies, introduce edible flowers gradually, as they may exacerbate allergies.

ANISE HYSSOP Both flowers and leaves have a subtle anise or licorice flavor.

ARUGULA Blossoms are small with dark centers and a peppery flavor much like the leaves. They range in color from white to yellow with dark purple streaks.

BACHELOR'S BUTTON Grassy in flavor, the petals are edible, but avoid the bitter calyx (the green part behind the petals).

BASIL Blossoms come in a variety of colors, from white to pink to lavender; flavor is similar to the leaves, but milder.

BEE BALM The red flowers have a minty flavor.

BORAGE Blossoms are a lovely blue hue, and they taste like cucumber.

CALENDULA A great flower for eating, calendula blossoms are peppery, tangy, and spicy—and their vibrant golden color adds dash to any dish.

CARNATION / DIANTHUS Petals are sweet, once trimmed away from the base. The blossoms taste like their sweet, perfumed aroma.

CHAMOMILE Small and daisylike, the flowers have a sweet flavor often used in tea. Ragweed allergy sufferers may be allergic to them as well.

CHERVIL Delicate blossoms have an anise-tinged flavor.

CHICORY Mildly bitter earthiness of chicory is evident in the petals and buds, which can be pickled.

CHRYSANTHEMUM A little bitter, mums come in a rainbow of colors and a range of flavors, from peppery to pungent. Use only the petals.

CILANTRO People either love these blossoms or hate them. The flowers share the grassy flavor of the herb. Use them fresh, as they lose their charm when heated.

To keep flowers fresh, place them on moist paper towels and refrigerate in an airtight container. Some will last up to ten days this way. Ice water can revitalize limp flowers.

CITRUS Citrus blossoms are sweet and highly scented. Use them frugally or they will overperfume a dish.

CLOVER Flowers are sweet with a hint of licorice.

DANDELION The blossoms themselves are surprisingly sweet and grassy. Young leaves are tasty, but stems are bitter. Toss petals into salad or stir buds into eggs.

DAYLILY Buds and flowers are sweet, edible raw or cooked. Even spent flowers add flavor to soup.

DILL Yellow dill flowers taste much like the herb's leaves.

Be sure you know your flowers before you serve them as part of a meal. Daylilies are edible, for example, but true lilies (such as tiger lilies or Easter lilies, for instance) are not. Violets and pansies are safely edible, but African violets are not. Don't let common names mislead you.

ENGLISH DAISY These aren't the best-tasting petals—they are somewhat bitter, but they look great, and they are totally safe if one were to eat them!

FENNEL Yellow fennel flowers are eye candy with a subtle licorice flavor, much like the herb itself.

FUCHSIA Tangy fuchsia flowers make a beautiful garnish.

GLADIOLUS Who knew? Although gladioli are bland, they can be stuffed, or their petals separated and arranged for an interesting salad garnish.

HIBISCUS Famously used in hibiscus tea, this beautiful flower has a vibrant cranberry flavor and can be used sparingly.

HOLLYHOCK Bland and vegetal in flavor, hollyhock blossoms make a showy, edible garnish.

JASMINE These super-fragrant blooms are used in tea; you can also use them in sweet dishes, but sparingly.

JOHNNY-JUMP-UP Adorable and delicious, the flowers have a subtle mint flavor great for salads, pastas, fruit dishes, and drinks.

LAVENDER Sweet, spicy, and perfumed, the flowers are a great addition to both savory and sweet dishes.

LEMON VERBENA The diminutive off-white blossoms are redolent of lemon—and great for teas and desserts.

LILAC The blooms are pungent, but the floral citrusy aroma translates to its flavor as well.

MARIGOLD The flower petals are all edible, but only the single petal varieties called signet marigolds taste good.

MINT The flowers are—no surprise—minty. Their intensity varies among varieties.

Cream of Dandelion Soup

There is a traditional soup in France, creme de pissenlits *(cream of dandelions), which balances dandelion's piquant bitterness with other savory flavors. It is delicious, combining the French* grandmère *and down-home Southern cooking. The traditional French recipe uses Dijon mustard. It adds some spicy depth, but it's optional.* SERVES 6 TO 8

- 2 pounds (about 6 cups) dandelion greens, trimmed and washed
- 1 tablespoon butter or olive oil
- 1 carrot, diced
- 2 large leeks, white and light parts only, washed and sliced
- 4 cups vegetable stock
- 2 ½ cups milk
- Salt and pepper to taste
- 1 tablespoon Dijon mustard (optional)
- Dandelion buds and/or flower petals for garnish

1. If using more mature or very bitter-tasting greens, blanch them in a pot of boiling salted water, then drain and squeeze out the excess water, chop, and set aside.

2. Heat butter or oil in a large pot over medium high heat, add greens, carrot, and leeks and cook, stirring often, for 15 minutes.

3. Add stock and simmer for about 15 minutes. Reduce heat to medium, whisk in milk, and cook, stirring frequently, until slightly thickened.

4. Puree mix in a tightly covered blender until smooth, taking care with the hot liquid. Season with salt and pepper, and add mustard if you like.

5. Serve in bowls and garnish with flowers or buds.

NASTURTIUM One of the most popular edible flowers, nasturtium blossoms are brilliantly colored with a sweet, floral flavor and a spicy pepper finish. The seed pod is a marvel of sweet and spicy. You can stuff the flowers, add the leaves to salads, and pickle the buds like capers.

OREGANO The flowers are a pretty, subtle version of the leaf.

PANSY The petals are bland in flavor, but if you eat the whole flower you get more taste.

RADISH Varying in color, radish flowers have a distinctive, peppery bite.

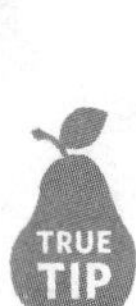

To learn more about biodynamic farming and gardening—a philosophy and practice concerned with the vitality of the soil in which all things grow, visit this website: *www.biodynamics.org*.

ROSE All roses are edible, with flavor more pronounced in darker varieties. Remove the petals from the white, bitter base for lovely color, texture, and a strongly perfumed flavor, perfect for floating in drinks, scattering across desserts, and making jams.

ROSEMARY Flowers taste like a milder version of the herb; nice as a garnish on dishes that incorporate rosemary.

SAGE Blossoms have a subtle flavor similar to the leaves.

SQUASH AND PUMPKIN Blossoms from both are wonderful vehicles for stuffing. Each has a slight squash flavor. Remove stamens before using.

SUNFLOWER Petals can be eaten, and the bud can be steamed like an artichoke.

VIOLETS Another famous edible flower, violets are floral, sweet, and beautiful as garnishes. Use the flowers in salads and to garnish desserts and drinks.

A basket of produce lands on the kitchen counter.... Look at this food. There are no ingredient labels, no health claims, nothing to read.... This is food, so fresh it's still alive, communicating with us by scent and color and taste.

—MICHAEL POLLAN, *IN DEFENSE OF FOOD*

Adding a Wild Touch to the Menu

Native Americans gathered and ate plants that most of us have never heard of. From agarita, alpine strawberry, American turk's cap lily, and arrow grass to white oak, wild calla, woolly milk vetch, and yellow wild indigo, their diets depended on native wild plants.

Now that knowledge has been all but lost. For many people today, wild plants are equivalent to pesky weeds.

Healthy for You

SEASONAL FORAGERS' FINDS

- **SPRING GREENS**
  Cattail stalks, dandelion, chickweed, chives, nettle, wild lettuce, violet leaves
- **SPRING FLOWERS & BERRIES**
  Redbud, mustard and rose family, violet, strawberry, gooseberry
- **SPRING ROOTS**
  Burdock, dandelion, wild parsnip
- **SUMMER HERBS**
  Clover flowers, horsetail tops, chamomile flowers, raspberry leaves, yarrow, bergamot
- **SUMMER FRUITS**
  Chokeberries, raspberries, mulberries, wild plum
- **SUMMER GREENS**
  Grape leaves, lamb's quarters, amaranth, wood sorrel
- **FALL ROOTS**
  Daylily, Jerusalem artichoke, marshmallow, burdock, wild parsnip
- **FALL GREENS**
  Purslane, watercress, dandelion
- **FALL NUTS**
  Hazelnut, pecan, hickory, acorn, walnut
- **FALL FRUITS**
  Grape, hawthorn, chokeberry, wintergreen, wild apples
- **WINTER GREENS**
  Chives, garlic mustard, watercress, thistle
- **WINTER ROOTS**
  Arrowhead, burdock, cattail, thistle
- **WINTER FRUITS**
  Bayberry, juniper berry, wintergreen berry, rose hips

Fortunately, expert foragers are keeping the tradition alive, and finding ever new ways to bring the remarkable flavors of wild plants into contemporary cooking. We can learn a great deal from them.

HOW TO START FORAGING "Nature is providing a whole abundant grocery store for us, and it's very easy for the gardener, or even someone who just goes on a weekend walk or bike ride, to find food," says herbalist Deborah Lee. She recommends introducing yourself to two or three plants a season, or a year, so as not to become overwhelmed. To help learn plant identification, Lee advises obtaining a copy of the Peterson *Field Guide to Edible Plants.* "Identify a plant, nibble on it a little bit, and figure out how to add it to a meal," says Lee. "Try chickweed, lamb's quarters (a kind of wild spinach), or violet leaves, for example. They're not much stronger tasting than lettuce." They add nutrients, fiber—and surprise—to a meal.

TRUE TIP

Dandelion is the quintessential wild plant whose possibilities have been forgotten: spring leaves, buds, and flowers are edible. And don't forget famous dandelion wine, made from the blooms.

Wild Spring Salad

An easy way to introduce wild things to friends and family is to add a few spring greens and flowers into a familiar tossed salad. Use a light dressing so the wild flavors come through. SERVES 4 TO 6

1 tablespoon olive oil
1 teaspoon balsamic vinegar
2 teaspoons lemon juice
1 bulb wild garlic (or 1 clove standard garlic), finely minced
Salt and pepper to taste
1 head butter lettuce
1 cup chickweed, stems and leaves
½ cup violet leaves
½ cup freshly picked violet flowers

1. Blend oil, vinegar, lemon juice, minced garlic, salt, and pepper.

2. Gently pick over, rinse, and pat dry lettuce, chickweed, and violet leaves.

3. Carefully pick over violet flowers, but do not rinse them. Hold back as you prepare the salad.

4. Just before serving, toss greens with dressing and garnish the salad with violet flowers.

Healthy for You

BEST PRACTICES WITH WILD FOODS

- Know what you are picking. Many edible plants have a poisonous lookalike. Once the edible plant has been definitively identified, take a tiny nibble, then wait for 30 minutes to observe any adverse reactions. As a general rule of thumb, if a plant has any red or purple on the leaves, leave it alone: About 90 percent of the time it will be toxic.
- Be extremely careful when collecting mushrooms. A novice can easily make serious mistakes.
- Know what part of the plant to pick. One may be safe to eat and another toxic. For example, elderberry blossoms and fruit are edible, but the leaves and branches are poisonous; early poke sprouts are good when properly cooked, but harmful later in the season.
- Just because animals eat a plant does not mean humans can eat it, too.
- Avoid plants in commercially fertilized areas. Some plants, such as lamb's quarters, absorb toxic levels of nitrates from commercial fertilizer. Also avoid collecting under power lines, in unfamiliar weed lots or lawns, or beside farmers' fields—all areas that may be sprayed with herbicides, pesticides, or defoliants.
- Avoid foraging on main roadsides. Plants may be sprayed with toxic chemicals and coated with exhaust from cars.
- Collect with consciousness. Rule of thumb: Never gather the first of anything you see. As foragers, we have a responsibility to maintain the habitat in which we collect, even to make it better.
- Take only what you need. Leave some for wildlife to forage and some to reproduce.
- Clean and sort gathered food in the field or woods. No cook wants a sink full of muddy dandelion greens, grass blades, and ants.
- Practice moderation. Wild edibles are powerful foods, and your system may need to adjust. Eating them may rid the body of toxins, but you want this beneficial cleansing to occur slowly.
- Combine wild foods, many of which have strong flavors, with family favorites. Add wild greens to soup, steam them with cabbage, or saute them with onions. Toss wild greens or flowers into a salad.

STEP

Eat Whole Foods

Fill your plate high with whole foods—fresh produce, whole grains, nuts, and seeds. Their fiber and essential nutrients play a beneficial role in the body's metabolic processes and in its defenses against cancer, heart disease, and common digestive ailments. In comparison, refined foods like white flour and granulated sugar are inert and lifeless, stripped of fiber, nutrients, and enzymes to provide a longer shelf life at the expense of flavor and nourishment.

WHAT IT MEANS

Unprocessed and Unrefined

Nutritionally complex whole foods provide a wide variety of benefits.

A potato chip is made of a potato, so it's a whole food, right? Not quite. A whole food has undergone very little processing before being consumed. Processing food removes important nutrients: The more refined the food, the fewer nutrients it contains.

The comparison in nutritional value between refined and unrefined wheat flour is a striking example of the disparity. Whole-grain wheat flour is made from the entire grain, including the bran, endosperm, and germ, rich in minerals like magnesium, zinc, iron, and the vitamins E, A, and B_6. "White" flour is a refined wheat flour that has been stripped of some of its most valuable nutrients, such as the vitamins E, A, and B, along with the fiber. The bran and the germ have been removed, leaving only the endosperm, the tissue around the embryo of the seed. In fact, one-half cup of unbleached white flour has no fiber, while one-half cup of whole wheat flour has eight grams, a significant difference. "Enriched" flour has some of the nutrients added back in, but not all: Fiber, enzymes, the bran and germ, and many vitamins and minerals are not returned.

Some people like to paint pictures or build a boat in the basement. Others get a tremendous pleasure out of the kitchen because cooking is just as creative and imaginative an activity as drawing, or woodcarving, or music.

—JULIA CHILD, *MASTERING THE ART OF FRENCH COOKING*

WHY IT MATTERS FOR YOU

Necessary Nutrients

Whole foods contain complex carbohydrates, fiber, and a host of other nutrients.

Whole foods—including fruits, vegetables, unrefined grains, nuts, and seeds—are the most healthful foods we can eat. Whole grains have been shown to reduce the risk of heart disease and cancer by providing essential nutrients like vitamins A and E and considerable amounts of fiber. Crucial nutrients necessary for health (and for the metabolism) are missing from refined food.

WHY IT MATTERS FOR EARTH

Processing and Packaging

More food handling means more environmental pollution.

Processed food requires more steps, increasing waste disposal, fuel emissions, and packaging. Packaging accounts for one-third of municipal solid waste. Plastics take up 32 percent of landfill space by volume and by weight; paper and paperboard take up 30.2 percent; glass takes up 2.2 percent; and aluminum takes up 2.4 percent.

Five of the six chemicals that generate the most hazardous waste, as ranked by the Environmental Protection Agency (EPA), are used in the plastics industry. Dioxin and 300 other organochlorines have been identified in the runoff from pulp bleaching in paper mills. Buying whole foods reduces packaging. When you do buy processed food, support companies whose plants practice bioconversion of by-products and waste into edible food.

HOW TO DO IT

A Big Step

Think of it as an adventure.

Don't expect to switch from refined to whole foods in one trip to the market—whole foods are a new world of edibles to explore. Take your time playing with these foods until you have built a repertoire of whole foods to replace the refined ones that you may rely on now.

If you bake, you can start by replacing some of the white flour with a whole-grain flour bit by bit, eventually aiming to use only whole-grain flours. Start by experimenting with new grains in your cooking, swapping white rice for brown rice or for other unmilled heirloom rices. Check the labels on all grain-based products you buy—bread, crackers, pasta—and look for the word "whole" at the top of the list of ingredients. This means that whole grains are being used.

Fiber

Impressive health claims are made about high-fiber diets. Reportedly, they may reduce incidences of colon and other cancers, lower cholesterol, reduce the rate of heart disease, and lower the blood sugar of diabetics.

Researchers speculate that a high-fiber diet reduces the risk of heart disease. When you eat fiber-rich carbohydrates, your blood sugar levels do not go as high, which slows down the release of insulin. (The more refined the carbohydrate, the more quickly our bodies turn it into glucose, and insulin levels rise to handle the sugar rush.) High levels of insulin are a factor in heart disease and diabetes. Under a doctor's supervision, diabetics on high-fiber diets can reduce the insulin they require. Lower insulin levels may also reduce cholesterol synthesis.

British physician Denis Burkitt reported in the early 1970s that Africans had significantly fewer cases of colon cancer and other diseases such as diverticular disease, and even had fewer varicose veins. He observed that the African diet was very high in fiber (60 or more grams a day), and that Africans had a "gut transit time" for the elimination of food waste that was one-third that of meat-eating Europeans with a low-fiber diet. Among other benefits (such as soft stools), the sped-up elimination of digested food on a high-fiber diet meant that poisons (intestinal bacteria) spent less time building up in the digestive tract, thereby possibly preventing digestive ailments, including constipation and, ultimately, colon cancer.

Burkitt's findings have been echoed by other scientists. A study at Memorial Sloan-Kettering Cancer Center found that a high-fiber diet could shrink precancerous

Healthy for You

FACTS ON FIBER

There are two kinds of fiber—soluble and insoluble—both found in plant foods such as grains, nuts, and seeds as well as in fruits and vegetables. Both are necessary for good health, and luckily most plant foods contain both kinds.

Insoluble fiber does not dissolve in water (the hull around grains is a good example of this). It works to balance the intestinal pH and to move bulk through the intestines, thereby limiting toxins in waste. Sources include greens, green beans, corn bran, seeds and nuts, wheat, and fruit and vegetable skins.

Soluble fiber, such as oat bran, becomes glutinous in contact with water. The fiber reduces the emptying time of the stomach so that sugar is released more slowly. This, in turn, lowers total cholesterol and LDL cholesterol. Sources include oat bran, flaxseed, fruits, vegetables, and psyllium husk.

growths of the colon. Researchers from around the world have found that people who eat a diet high in fiber have lower cancer rates overall.

HOW MUCH FIBER?

The recommended daily allowance for fiber is 20 to 30 grams. Some health practitioners recommend that people eat as much as 60 grams a day. If you decide to increase your fiber intake, make sure you do it slowly and drink a lot of water. Consuming too much fiber too quickly can cause constipation, just as too little fiber can.

Sugar

Next to "white" flour, the other most refined food in the American diet is sugar. The average American eats 14 pounds of sweeteners a year.

"Pure" refined sugar made its debut in 1812, when a chemist invented a method of extracting the juice from sugarcane and the sugar beet, leaving the bulk and fiber behind. To make granulated sugar as we know it, this juice is then purified, filtered, concentrated, and boiled down until the syrup crystallizes. The resulting product is 99.9 percent sugar crystals, the ultimate in a refined carbohydrate. Refined sugars include white table sugar, turbinado (raw sugar that has been refined and cleaned), brown sugar (essentially the same as white sugar, with the addition of a small amount of molasses or caramel color), confectioners' sugar (sugar plus cornstarch), and corn syrup, produced from cornstarch. Glucose (dextrose), fructose, maltose, and lactose are also considered sugars.

Contrary to common belief, sugar has not been found to cause either hyperactivity in children (this is still controversial) or diabetes. However, obesity can cause diabetes, and eating too many refined foods can cause obesity. Refined carbohydrates are full of empty calories, which lack nutritional value. "Refined dietary sugars

Fiber Content of Foods

FOOD	SERVING SIZE	FIBER (GRAMS)
Barley, pearl	1 cup cooked	6
Buckwheat flour	1 cup	12
Cornmeal	1 cup	9
Millet	1 cup cooked	3
Oats	1 cup cooked	4
Rice, brown	1 cup cooked	4
Rice, brown	1 cup cooked	7
Rye	1 cup flour	29
Wheat, whole	1 cup flour	14
Black beans	1 cup cooked	14
Black-eyed peas	1 cup cooked	12
Garbanzo beans	1 cup cooked	10
Great Northern beans	1 cup cooked	12
Kidney beans	1 cup cooked	12
Lentils	1 cup cooked	16
Mung beans	1 cup cooked	15

FOOD	SERVING SIZE	FIBER (GRAMS)
Navy beans	1 cup cooked	16
Peas	1 cup cooked	16
Pinto beans	1 cup cooked	15
Soybeans	1 cup cooked	10
Almonds	1 cup	15
Cashews	1 cup	4
Filberts	1 cup	9
Peanuts	1 cup	12
Pecans	1 cup halves	8
Pumpkin seeds	1 cup	22
Walnuts	1 cup	6
Artichoke	1 medium	5
Asparagus	1 cup	5
Beans, snap	1 cup cooked	4
Broccoli	1 cup cooked	5
Brussels sprouts	1 cup cooked	6
Cauliflower	1 cup cooked	4
Corn	1 cup cooked	4

STEP 6

EAT WHOLE FOODS

Fiber Content of Foods *(continued)*

FOOD	SERVING SIZE	FIBER (GRAMS)
Eggplant	1 cup cooked	2
Kohlrabi	1 cup cooked	3
Okra	1 cup cooked	4
Parsnips	1 cup cooked	3
Peas, edible pods	1 cup	4
Potato	1 cooked	4
Pumpkin	1 cup	4
Spinach	1 cup raw	1
Squash (yellow summer)	1 cup cooked	4
Squash (zucchini)	1 cup cooked	4
Squash (acorn)	1 cup cooked	6
Squash (butternut)	1 cup cooked	5
Sweet potato	1 cup cooked	8
Turnip	1 cup cooked	4

FOOD	SERVING SIZE	FIBER (GRAMS)
Apple, raw whole	1 medium	4
Apricots	2	2
Avocado	1 medium	8
Banana	1 medium	3
Blueberries	½ cup	2
Cherries	1 cup	3
Grapefruit	½ medium	2
Mango	1	4
Nectarine	1	2
Orange	1 medium	3
Papaya	½	3
Peach	1 medium	2
Pear	1 medium	4
Plum	1 medium	1
Pomegranate	1	1
Raspberries	½ cup	3
Strawberries	½ cup	3
Tangerine	1 medium	1
Watermelon	1 cup	.5

Source: USDA

almost always turn into fats," warns Udo Erasmus, author of *Fats That Heal and Fats That Kill*. "Our body stores excess glucose from times of feasting—as fat—for use in future times of famine," he explains.

HEALTHY SUGARS? Are any sweeteners healthier than others? A common point that many nutritionists make is that all carbohydrates, which are made up of basic sugar units such as glucose or fructose, act the same way in our bodies. So it doesn't matter if we eat sugar or rice syrup, the body will react the same way to both. But an important issue left out of this argument is that foods containing less refined sugars, such as blackstrap molasses, have retained much of their nutritional value. It is precisely those nutrients that may help the body handle the rise in glucose and the subsequent release of insulin. "Refined sugars need no digestion and are absorbed rapidly. They lack the co-factors, and our bodies cannot burn them properly," Erasmus writes.

Refined sugars can actually leach nutrients from the body. High-fructose corn syrup is a popular alternative to sugar and is found in everything from soda to peanut butter. It has been determined, however, that this refined sweetener depletes chromium, a mineral essential to the body's ability to use and digest sugar properly. When corn syrup is eaten in conjunction with sugar (having soda and cake together, for instance), chromium depletion is further aggravated. This can lead to an increase in triglycerides and blood cholesterol—increases that factor into our risk for diabetes and heart disease.

The New Foragers: Shopping for Whole Foods

No matter where you live in the country, there are ways to find whole, unprocessed, and locally grown organic food. In fact, whole foods are so flavorful and appealing, they are increasingly in demand and available; however, unprocessed and organic products can't be called mainstream. You may have to become something of a modern forager to find a steady and abundant supply.

Though you will probably be able to locate at least a few foods with minimal processing and additives in just about any supermarket, a more plentiful supply of organic foods—particularly high-quality fruits and vegetables—is found at health food stores, natural food stores, green supermarkets, food co-ops, farmers' markets, local farms, and through mail order and online, to name a few sources.

A successful and common combination of approaches for acquiring fresh, whole food is to visit a supermarket or health food store once a week, order from a food co-op once a month, and find a source of local and organic produce. That can be the biggest challenge, but farmers' markets are popping up everywhere. Eventually, your appreciation of the flavor of local, organic fresh food will be the only motivation you will need to make the extra effort to find it.

CONVENTIONAL STORES A big shift has taken place in mainstream supermarkets. In 1992 only 12 percent of senior supermarket managers felt that offering "natural" products was important; today almost every supermarket chain offers a robust natural foods selection. Urban environments have entire supermarkets devoted to natural foods. Now if we could just inspire supermarkets to buy from local farmers!

These new green supermarkets—which make a business of offering a large selection of whole food, often organic—are doing a booming business. Mainstream supermarkets aren't far behind with some, such as Safeway, ramping up by selling local produce. To find green supermarkets, however, you usually need to live near a big city or large town. For those of us who don't, local health food stores, farmers' markets, and even local farms and gardens are all good options.

HEALTH FOOD STORES The food found in health food stores—or in the "natural" food section of supermarket chains—rarely contains additives. The food is often whole and organic, but not always. In fact, many of the bakery items and pasta will be made with white flour. You still need to read all the labels. That being said, however, health food stores are excellent sources for soy products such as tofu; organic dairy, including yogurt and cheese;

Healthy for You

THE GLYCEMIC INDEX

The glycemic index (GI) ranks foods according to how much they raise blood sugar levels when eaten. Foods with a low GI are slowly digested and absorbed, producing gradual rises in blood sugar levels.

How high your blood glucose rises depends on the quantity and quality of carbo-hydrates consumed. The glycemic load combines both measures into one number. Eating at least one low-GI meal a day will keep your blood glucose low and give you a balanced amount of carbs, fats, and proteins.

Proteins are low on the glycemic index; candy and white bread are high. For a database of foods and how they stack up on the glycemic index, visit *www.glycemicindex.com.*

FOOD	CARBOHYDRATES	GLYCEMIC INDEX	GLYCEMIC LOAD
12 oz. cola drink	26 grams	63	36.4
fresh apple (medium)	21 grams	54	11.3
2 tbsp. agave nectar	32 grams	30	9.6

eggs from free-range hens; locally grown organic produce and meats; whole-grain cereals; tomato or spinach whole-wheat wraps and Mexican food wrappers such as tortillas; and whole-food snacks, nuts and seeds, dried fruits, and, for special occasions, even candy without food dyes. As with green supermarkets, health food stores tend to stock the greenest cleaning products available. As a general rule, the smaller the health food store, the more it will tend to carry primarily snacks and vitamins.

MAIL-ORDER CATALOGS A great deal of whole, organic food can be bought through the mail—everything from dairy products like cheese, to fresh bread, to weekly deliveries of organic produce baskets and organic meats as well as bulk nuts and seeds, specialty grain and flours, and unrefined sugars. There are hundreds of mail-order catalogs. Buying family groceries through the mail can open up an entire array of healthful options for those who

Shopping & Saving

HOW TO READ NUTRITION LABELS

The FDA is responsible for assuring that food sold in the U.S. is "safe, wholesome and appropriately labeled." The Nutrition Labeling and Education Act requires foods under FDA jurisdiction to bear nutrition labeling and requires food labels bearing nutrient content claims and health claims to comply with specific requirements. Of the three ways the FDA describes its responsibility to the food system—"safe, wholesome, and appropriately labeled"—"wholesome" is the least well defined. Is a hydrogenated oil wholesome? Or sweeteners made from synthetic chemicals?
The FDA apparently thinks so; we disagree. Fortunately, in most cases, good label reading will help you steer clear of undesirable foods.

have difficulty finding local outlets for wholesome, freshly picked organic foods or ranch-raised meats. Weekly shipments can be ordered for overnight delivery. Usually the produce is picked the morning it is shipped.

Packaged organic food is readily available through the mail too. In fact, some co-op wholesalers will even ship orders with no minimum, via UPS, for those who don't want to start a buying club. To explore sources near or far, visit the Local Harvest website: *www.localharvest.org.*

Finding Whole Foods in Grocery Stores

In the following guide, food product categories are listed alphabetically. Within most categories you will find the following sections:

BEST CHOICE Identifies the product closest to a whole food with the fewest additives; however, for some foods there are no good choices and "None" is recommended. To avoid redundancy, we do not state "organic" for every "best choice," but we are recommending certified organic whenever possible.

ALERT Lists additives or treatments of possible concern.

CONCERNS, GENERAL CONCERNS, SPECIAL CONCERNS Further comments about the product category.

If you shop in conventional stores and want to buy whole foods, read ingredients labels for every food product you buy. Only the label will tell the truth about the food you are buying. If the ingredients are unappealing, move on to the labels of similar products until you find a good choice. With very few exceptions, there is a whole-food choice for every food product category. And don't be fooled by claims on the package: Sometimes the "blueberry" waffles contain no blueberries.

Baked Goods and Baking Supplies

Breads, Crackers, and Flours

BEST CHOICE Look for whole-grain breads and crackers such as whole wheat, corn, oats, barley, rice, amaranth, and rye. Make sure the words "whole wheat" are on ingredient labels for wheat products. Look for whole-grain baked goods with the fewest ingredients on the label: for example, whole wheat, water, yeast, and salt.

ALERT Many breads and crackers are made with refined

Cooking & Eating

MEET WHITE WHOLE-WHEAT FLOUR

Consider this your "trainer" whole wheat flour! The name is a little confusing, but the flour is amazing. White wheat is a naturally occurring albino variety of wheat, and when it is turned into whole wheat flour it doesn't have the nuttier taste or graininess of the common whole wheat flour (made from red wheat) we are accustomed to. White whole-wheat flour has the same nutritional and fiber benefits of red whole wheat, but since it doesn't have the same tannins and phenolic acid found in the outer bran of red wheat, it is both lighter in color and milder in flavor. Baked goods made with white whole-wheat flour are nearly indistinguishable from those prepared with refined white flour, but the difference in fiber and nutrients is substantial. White whole-wheat flour is available from America's oldest flour company, King Arthur Flour.

flour, sugar, excessive salt, hydrogenated oils, artificial colors and flavors, dough conditioners, and preservatives.

SPECIAL CONCERNS "Enriched flour" means that the flour has been stripped of much of its nutritional value, and vitamins have been added back in, in an attempt to compensate. The best flour is milled at home or freshly milled at a store. The reason is that the natural oils in freshly milled flour will not be rancid. If you buy packaged flour, buy small amounts at a time, and store in the freezer. Make sure to buy whole-grain flour—whole wheat, oat, brown rice, corn. White flour is not a whole-grain flour. Unbleached white flour with germ means that the wheat germ has been removed from the grain and then replaced. However, when wheat germ is exposed to air, its nutritional value diminishes considerably, and the oils in the germ can become rancid.

OTHER CONCERNS Read ingredient labels particularly carefully for baked goods such as boxed coffee cakes and doughnuts, as they often contain many additives. Baking mixes can contain hydrogenated oils, sugar, BHT, artificial color, artificial flavor, and preservatives. Breakfast toaster pastries can contain significant amounts of artificial colors and flavors. Highly seasoned products, such as croutons, may have a high fat content, and artificial flavors.

Baking Powder

BEST CHOICE Baking powder without sodium aluminum sulfate.

GENERAL CONCERNS Sodium aluminum sulfate: Although baking powder is not a major source of aluminum intake, and although aluminum has not been proven to cause Alzheimer's disease, high levels of aluminum have been found in the brains of people with Alzheimer's, so it's prudent to avoid aluminum whenever possible.

NOTE: Low-sodium baking powder uses potassium bicarbonate instead of sodium bicarbonate.

Sugar and Sweeteners

BEST CHOICES Maple syrup, honey, unrefined sugar, molasses, rice syrup, date sugar, barley malt, stevia, concentrated fruit juice.

NOTE: The color of honey has to do with the flowers from which the bees harvested the nectar and does not indicate nutritional content. However, the darker the color, the more pungent the flavor.

Whole Wheat Buttermilk Pancakes

If the words "whole wheat pancakes" bring to mind a plate of dense and hockey-puck-heavy flapjacks, you're in for a surprise. By using white whole-wheat flour in this recipe, you get all the goodness of whole grains in a light, flavorful pancake that is filling, yet so light it practically hovers above the plate. SERVES 3 TO 4

- 1 cup white whole-wheat flour
- ½ teaspoon baking powder
- ¼ teaspoon baking soda
- ¼ cup unrefined sugar
- ¼ teaspoon salt
- 1 ¾ cups organic buttermilk (or 1 cup yogurt and ¾ cup milk)
- 1 large free-range egg, lightly beaten
- 1 tablespoon melted butter
- Oil or butter for the pan

1. Stir all dry ingredients together in a large bowl, then add wet ingredients.

2. Stir lightly until just combined, leaving some lumps. Overbeating will result in tough pancakes.

3. Brush skillet with oil or butter and heat on medium until a droplet of water sizzles. Pour batter into pan and cook until small bubbles form. Flip, cook, and remove to a warm plate.

ALERT Minute amounts of lead are found in some maple syrup. The cause is the lead solder found in older maple sugaring equipment. The syrup with the highest lead contamination seems to be from small hobby operations where the sap can sit in a tank for a day or two. Commercial operations move sap very fast, so their syrups are less likely to pick up lead.

Vanilla Extract

BEST CHOICE Real vanilla flavoring, extracted from whole vanilla bean in either alcohol or water (rather than artificial flavor).
ALERT Vanillin, an artificial flavor.
GENERAL CONCERNS Always double-check the vanilla before buying it in bulk; if it has a pungent alcohol smell, it has turned bad. All liquid vanilla has alcohol in it, so even with fresh vanilla there is an alcohol smell, but with bad vanilla, the smell will be strong. Pure vanilla extract may contain glycerin, propylene glycol, sugar dextrose, or corn syrup, and the content of ethyl alcohol is not less than 35 percent by volume. "Vanilla flavoring" means extract with less than 35 percent alcohol.

Beverages

Coffee

BEST CHOICE Preferably organic coffee from shade-grown beans. Look for the Fair Trade Certified label, which ensures that farmers are being paid fair wages for their labor.
GENERAL CONCERNS There are four ways to decaffeinate coffee. One way is the Swiss water-processed method, using pure water; this is the purest method available. Two chemical methods of decaffeination use methylene chloride and ethyl acetate, solvents approved for use in the United States by the FDA. Methylene chloride is a carcinogen. Ethyl acetate does not pose risk to the consumer. The fourth method of decaffeination is water and carbon dioxide. If the label says "naturally decaffeinated," it was decaffeinated by either the Swiss water-processed method or the water and carbon dioxide method. Decaffeinated coffee manufactured in the U.S. is mostly done through water processing.

Avoid bleached-paper filters, which may contain small amounts of dioxin. Buy unbleached coffee filters or a reusable gold filter instead.
NOTE: You can help protect migratory birds' winter home habitat by buying coffee made from shade-grown beans. Usually organic, the coffee comes from farms that use the traditional

Simple Stewardship

BOTTLED WATER

In the United States last year, more than 22 billion empty plastic bottles were tossed into the trash. That is a lot of waste. Then there are the 1.5 million barrels of oil used to produce those bottles—enough petroleum to power 100,000 automobiles for an entire year.

Plastic is not healthy for our planet, or for you either. The full range of plastic's effects on the human body is not yet known, but studies into the different kinds of plastic are making it look as if none are really safe, and the list of harmful ones is growing. Endocrine disrupters, which resemble chemical hormones, have been found to cause genetic damage in developing fetuses and children. These chemicals have also been found to cause hormone-related cancers, such as breast cancer, in animals, and can leach from the plastic packaging into food and liquid. For a while the commonly used water bottle (plastic # 1) was considered safe, but no longer.

Bisphenol-A is one of the more well-known hormone-disrupting chemicals considered potentially harmful to human health and the environment. Scratched and worn polycarbonate bottles (plastic #7) will leach this chemical into liquids, and a movement is afoot to ban this material. For more information, visit *www.bisphenolafree.org.*

Check out the stainless steel water bottles on the market now. And don't let the "steel" part bother you—these are not the plain silver water bottles Grandpa used for camping! Make the switch that will protect your health and the environment.

under-tree growing style, rather than the more recent, pesticide-intensive, sun-grown method that destroys bird habitats. Shade-grown coffee provides habitats for migratory birds in Central and South America and Indonesia, as well as providing the fuller flavor of beans that have been slowly ripened.

Teas and Infusions

BEST CHOICE Loose leaves, herbs.
GENERAL CONCERNS When possible, buy tea bags made with unbleached cotton or paper.

NOTE: As with decaffeinated coffee, choose "naturally decaffeinated" tea.

Soda

BEST CHOICE Juice mixed with seltzer and only natural flavors.
GENERAL CONCERNS Commonly found additives: artificial color, artificial flavor, corn syrup, sugar, aspartame (NutraSweet or Equal), caffeine.
OTHER CONCERNS The sugar content of sodas can be a staggering 10 teaspoons per 12-ounce can. Even some "natural" sodas contain fructose as a sweetener.

Instant Hot Chocolate or Cocoa

BEST CHOICE Whole cocoa bought in bulk or large tin.
ALERT Artificial flavors, artificial dyes, preservatives, hydrogenated oils.
NOTE: Most supermarkets do not carry whole-food instant cocoa. Ask the manager to stock it, or look for it at your health food store. Since cocoa is not naturally sweet, you may want to sweeten the cocoa at home with a whole-food sweetener.

Syrups (Chocolate)

BEST CHOICE None.

Bottled Water

GENERAL CONCERNS The FDA defines bottled water as water that is sealed in bottles or other containers; this does not include mineral water or soda water. Bottled water must meet FDA regulations for trihalomethane, chloroform, and organic compounds. In addition, bottled water must meet standards of chemical quality and must not contain chemical substances and excess metals.

Juice

BEST CHOICE 100 percent freshly squeezed.
ALERT Watch out for added sugar. Look for a label that says "100 percent juice."

Frozen Juice Concentrates

BEST CHOICE 100 percent pure juice.
ALERT A product label should read "no added sugar" if it is made from concentrate; sweeteners such as aspartame (brand names NutraSweet, Equal) should be avoided.

Reconstituted Juice

ALERT If any water is added in excess of the amount of water needed to reconstitute the ingredient to single strength, the word "water" has to be listed among the ingredients.

Juice in Bottles, Aseptic Packaging, or Cans

BEST CHOICE 100 percent fruit juice.
ALERT Watch out for NutraSweet or Equal (aspartame).

Canned Goods

GENERAL CONCERNS Avoid canned food and drinks until there are labels with information about whether or not the cans are lined with plastic or contain lead. Canned fruits and vegetables are not as nutritious as fresh or frozen; cans that are lined in plastic can leach hormone-disrupting materials into food. Read canned soup lebels carefully, as some contain partially hydrogenated oils, sugar, sulfites, flavor enhancers, preservatives, and monosodium glutamate.

Baby Foods

BEST CHOICE Any plain baby food sold in glass jars, such as peaches, peas, carrots; plain, boxed whole-grain cereals. In choosing baby food it is desirable to buy products certified organic.
ALERT Avoid combo baby foods such as "chicken and pasta" or "apples and yogurt"; they are more likely to contain sugar, cornstarch, salt, or rice starch. Avoid baby food "desserts," very likely to contain sugar.
NOTE: The best solutions are your own purees of organic veggies and fruits.

Canned Tomatoes (see Canned Goods, above)

BEST CHOICE Tomatoes, tomato juice, pulp (salt, citric acid).
ALERT Hydrogenated oils. Most packers of tomato products effectively trim off, sort out, and discard rotten tomatoes; however, some mix rotten tomato products in with the healthy. The FDA defines these products as adulterated, but, since some slip through inspection, people with mold allergies should be particularly cautious about using canned tomato products.

Condiments, Dressings, Spreads

GENERAL CONCERNS When buying barbecue sauce, chili sauce, ketchup, and other condiments, read labels to avoid hydrogenated oils, preservatives, and artificial colors and flavors.

Mayonnaise

BEST CHOICE Substitute yogurt or another low-fat alternative. Otherwise choose a mayonnaise with only eggs, oil, and seasonings.
ALERT Partially hydrogenated oils, preservatives.
OTHER CONCERNS High fat content.

Oils

BEST CHOICE Look for oils labeled "expeller-pressed," "mechanically pressed," or, for olive oil, "cold-pressed." These oils have been extracted from the seed mechanically, as opposed to chemically. Another term for mechanically expressed oil is "unrefined."

SNAPSHOT **DAVID S. LUDWIG**

"The Atkins diet tries to get rid of all carbohydrates. You don't have to go to this extreme if you pay attention to the glycemic index and choose low-GI carbs."

Cambridge, Massachusetts

Pediatric endocrinologist

Founding Director, Optimal Weight for Life, Boston Children's Hospital

Dubbed an "obesity warrior" by *Time* magazine, David Ludwig is an Associate Professor in Pediatrics at Harvard Medical School. His research focuses on the effects of dietary composition on hormones, metabolism, and body weight regulation. Dr. Ludwig has fought for fundamental policy changes to restrict food advertising directed at young children, to improve quality of school nutrition programs, and to increase insurance reimbursement for obesity prevention and treatment programs. He also has developed a low glycemic diet—one that decreases the surge in blood sugar after meals—for the treatment of obesity and prevention of type-2 diabetes.

ALERT Solvent extraction is a chemical method of extracting oil from seeds. Hexane is the most common chemical used in solvent extraction. Oils obtained through this process are considered to be refined oils. "Refined" oils may include anti-clouding agents, BHT, BHA, and propyl gallate.

OTHER CONCERNS The term "cold-pressed" oil is misleading, since every oil (except olive oil, which can truly be cold-pressed) requires a temperature extraction level that seldom falls below 140° to 160°F. The high temperature required, however, is not believed to result in a loss of nutrients or flavor. "Refined" oil is also often stripped of oil's naturally occurring vitamin E, which can act as a natural preventative against rancidity. The "best choice" oils contain naturally occurring vitamin E.

Olive Oil

Because olive oil comes from the soft pulp of the fruit rather than from a seed, it needs no high-pressure extraction. Olives are crushed in a mill that breaks the pulp but not the pits. The first extraction is a gentle pressing that does not heat the oil much beyond room temperature. The oil is then separated from the olive water. Oil obtained from this first pressing is the only oil that can be called "virgin olive oil."

Virgin olive oil comes in three grades: extra-virgin, fine virgin, and plain virgin. The differences are solely those of taste and acidity, with plain virgin having the highest acid content and extra-virgin having the lowest.

"Pure" olive oil is still 100 percent olive oil, but it is not virgin. In other words, pure olive oil is extracted from second pressings, which require higher temperatures for extraction, reducing nutrient content, or solvent extraction.

Olives (Black)

BEST CHOICE Olives in water, salt, or brine (ferrous glucanate, iron, used to retain color).
ALERT Preservatives, salt.

Olives (Green)

BEST CHOICE Olives in water, salt, sorbic acid.
ALERT Thickening agents, preservatives, salt.

Jams and Jellies

BEST CHOICE Fruit (pectin, citric acid), no added sugar.

Pickles and Relishes

BEST CHOICE Cucumbers, peppers (salt or brine).
ALERT Salt, sulfiting agents, artificial colors.
NOTE: You have to look hard for pickles without artificial colors. If there are no acceptable brands in the traditional pickle aisle of your supermarket, try the dairy section or look elsewhere in the store for "kosher" dills, which are usually not dyed.

Salad Dressing

BEST CHOICE Oil, vinegar, spices, vegetables such as onions.

Vinegar (Distilled, Red/White Wine, Balsamic, Cider Vinegar)

BEST CHOICE 100 percent vinegar.
ALERT Sulfiting agents, for those who are allergic. Read the entire label scrupulously—some labels on balsamic vinegar, we discovered, listed sulfites in an obscure location.

The olive tree is surely the richest gift of Heaven.

—THOMAS JEFFERSON

Dairy Products

GENERAL CONCERNS One of the most controversial aspects of milk production is the use of rBGH, or recombinant bovine growth hormone (also called rBST). A bioengineered drug, rBGH is given to cows to increase milk production. Because of consumer and farmer dissatisfaction, rBGH is now used minimally. In fact, the New England dairy industry will be "rBST-free" by the end of summer 2009.

This controversial drug is widely misunderstood by the public. It is often assumed that the injection of this hormone into dairy cows results in its presence in the milk. In fact, what happens is that the drug stimulates the cows to overproduce the bovine insulin-like growth factor 1 (IGF-1), which many researchers believe is then absorbed into the human body. The problem is that too much IGF-1 can promote the overgrowth of cells, including those that are cancerous.

OTHER CONCERNS When a coloring has been added to butter, cheese, or ice cream, it does not need to be declared in the ingredients list unless it is a color additive that has special safety restrictions. Blue cheese often has blue and green dyes in it, for example, and blue and green dyes are often used to mask any yellowing in the curd of other dairy products. The FDA recommends voluntary declaration of all coloring.

Dairy ingredients are often bleached with benzoyl peroxide or a mixture of benzoyl peroxide with potassium alum, calcium sulfate, and magnesium carbonate.

The FDA allows residues of PCB concentrations in dairy products up to 1.5 parts per million.

Consider trying quark cheese, named for the German term for curds. It is a soft white cheese with a slightly acidic taste and smooth, spreadable texture. It is low in fat, sodium, and calories and derives only 30 percent of its calories from fat. Use it as a substitute for sour cream, cream cheese, Neufchatel cheese, ricotta, and cottage cheese. Choose freshly made quark, since its shelf life is about 14 days from manufacture.

Low-Fat Dairy Products

Some foods labeled "light," "low-fat," or "nonfat" contain more stabilizers, preservatives, and artificial flavors than their traditional counterparts. This is particularly true for foods labeled "nonfat."

Cottage cheese and yogurt products are examples of foods where the low-fat version can be as whole as the full-fat version, but the nonfat version has lots of preservatives and flavorings. Look for low-fat dairy products that do not contain chemical additives.

Butter

BEST CHOICES Organic salted or unsalted.

ALERT Saturated fat. Use sparingly. Butter can have added ingredients that are not required to be on the label, such as preservatives, flavor, sweeteners, and dyes.

NOTE: For the purest butter, buy from a dairy that doesn't use either rBST or additives.

Cheese

BEST CHOICE Low-fat cheese containing milk, cream, salt, rennet, cheese cultures.

ALERT Corn syrup, preservatives, sugar, food starch, artificial colors. Processed "cheese foods," processed cheeses, and "American" cheeses are likely to contain corn syrup, preservatives, and hydrogenated oils. Some cottage cheeses also contain sugar and food starches.

NOTE: As a rule of thumb, the harder cheeses have less fat content than the softer cheeses.

Chocolate Milk

BEST CHOICE Low-fat milk, cocoa, with whole-food sweetener such as Sucanat.

ALERT Sugar, corn syrup, artificial flavors and colors, preservatives.

Condensed or Evaporated Milk

BEST CHOICE None.

ALERT The processing causes a significant reduction of nutritional value.

Sweetened Condensed Milk

BEST CHOICE None.

ALERT Sugar, corn syrup, preservatives. The processing causes a significant reduction of nutritional value.

Cottage Cheese

BEST CHOICE Low-fat.

OTHER CONCERNS Cottage cheese with premixed fruit can have sugar, high-fructose corn syrup, aspartame (NutraSweet, Equal).

Cream Cheese

BEST CHOICE Low-fat.

ALERT "Light," "fat-free," or "soft" cream cheese tends to have more additives, preservatives, and artificial flavors.

Dried Milk

BEST CHOICE Organic dried or organic powdered milk.
ALERT Added vitamins, emulsifiers, preservatives; processing significantly reduces nutritional value.

Ice Cream and Frozen Yogurt

BEST CHOICE Low-fat ice cream and yogurts; fruit sorbet as a more healthful substitute.
OTHER CONCERNS Among traditional ice cream and frozen yogurt brands there is a wide range, from great whole-food choices containing just the essential ingredients—cream and sugar—to those containing many additives, large amounts of sugar or aspartame (NutraSweet, Equal), and preservatives.

Instant Coffee Creamers, Nondairy Creamers

BEST CHOICE None.
ALERT Corn syrup solids, partially hydrogenated oils, artificial flavor, preservatives; contains casinine, a milk product; fats.

Margarine

BEST CHOICE None.
ALERT Hydrogenated or partially hydrogenated oils.

Milk

BEST CHOICE 100 percent pasteurized low-fat cow's or goat's milk. An additive commonly found in milk is Vitamin D_3, a necessary nutrient added to milk.
OTHER CONCERNS Milk is a common allergen and has a high fat content. Choose low-fat and rBST-free milk whenever possible.

Sour Cream

BEST CHOICE Cultured cream, whey, enzymes.
ALERT Don't choose a substitute.
OTHER CONCERNS See Cream Cheese.

Yogurt

BEST CHOICE Yogurt containing milk (preferably skim), yogurt cultures, whole fruit, fruit juice sweetener.
ALERT Yogurts range widely from those containing milk, yogurt cultures, and plain fruit or fruit juices, to yogurts containing many additives and sugar.

Eggs

BEST CHOICE Eggs from free-range hens raised on organic feed and not treated with antibiotics.
ALERT All eggs should be cooked thoroughly, as the deadly bacterium

Shopping & Saving

WELL BREAD: READING THE LABELS

Don't judge a loaf by its color. Just because bread is brown doesn't mean it's more nutritious.

Sad to say, many breads wear a nutritious-looking disguise, achieved simply by adding coloring. To find out if a brown bread is really more nutritious, be a label sleuth.

- **WHEAT FLOUR** A blend of mostly white flour with some whole wheat flour.
- **WHOLE WHEAT FLOUR** Look for "whole wheat flour" or "100 percent whole wheat"—it should be first on the label.
- **ENRICHED FLOUR** White flour with a few—but far from all—nutrients added back after the refining process removed them.
- **BLEACHED FLOUR** White flour chemically treated to be whiter and brighter.

Salmonella enteritidis is found in raw eggs. PCBs have been found in eggs (FDA limit is 0.3 part per million). Eggs do not have to be dated if they have not been graded by the USDA; they do not have to be graded unless they come from a farm of more than 3,000 hens or a producer selling eggs from more than one farm.

Dried Foods and Seasonings

GENERAL CONCERNS Read labels carefully. You will find additives in unexpected places. Chili spice powder, for example, can contain sulfites; applesauce can contain artificial colors and even hydrogenated oils.

Cereal

BEST CHOICE Whole grains such as wheat, corn, or oats, without sweetener, or sweetened with whole foods sweetener.

GENERAL CONCERNS Sugar, corn syrup, artificial colors, partially hydrogenated oils, aspartame, artificial flavors, preservatives; BHT added to cereal.

NOTE: "Puffed" cereal is the least nutritious because high temperatures used to puff the grain kernel destroy vitamins and minerals in the process.

ALERT Most granolas contain a lot of oil, so they should be stored in a well-sealed container and refrigerated to keep oils from going rancid.

Healthy for You

THREE QUICK-COOKING GRAINS

QUINOA

Light and chewy, quinoa (pronounced KEEN-wah) is an ancient grain from the Andes that has an extraordinary protein content; in fact, it provides a complete protein. It is also a great source of iron and has a host of other wonderful nutritious elements. When quinoa is cooked, the crunchy germ rings separate slightly from the round creamy seed so they look like little ringed planets. The result is an intriguing contrast of texture and an addictive flavor that is at once sweet, nutty, and a little grassy. Quinoa needs to be rinsed first to remove the bitter, naturally occurring saponins. To make steamed quinoa, the grain-to-water ratio is 1:2.

MILLET

In the U.S., millet is probably eaten more by pet birds than by people. But in the rest of the world millet is known as a delicious, nutritious, quick-cooking staple. Millet is one of the smallest of the common grains, yet its nearly complete protein has more iron than many other cereal grains. When steamed with a lesser amount of water, millet puffs up like airy couscous; when cooked with more water, it has a polenta-like consistency. For fluffy millet, the grain-to-water ratio is 1:2; for polenta-like millet, the ratio is 1:3. Millet responds well if you toast it first, then rinse and cook it.

TEFF

Teff, another ancient grain, is a traditional Ethiopian staple with a sweet, dark, and malty flavor. It's a rich source of minerals but stands out for its calcium and iron content. An eight-ounce serving of teff provides 32 percent of the RDA for calcium and 80 percent for iron. Teff can be used in many different ways—in Ethiopia it is used to make the flatbread *injera*. Use it as you would barley or millet, or in place of cornmeal for polenta. The grain-to-water ratio is 1:3.

Herbs

GENERAL CONCERNS Ask your health food stores how quick the turnover is for the dried herbs sold in bulk. Quick turnovers offer you a better chance of buying a fresh product. Smell the herbs to check for staleness. Air and light destroy an herb's or spice's freshness; therefore it is best to buy the herb in its whole-leaf state, since crumbling the herb releases the essential oils that give the herb its flavor. The same goes for spices: Buy them whole and grind them in small batches.
ALERT Ask your store manager to label irradiated herbs.

Salt

BEST CHOICE Sea salt made from evaporated seawater, with added iodine (and dextrose to stabilize the iodine).
GENERAL CONCERNS Although purists would not agree that iodized sea salt is the best choice, iodine helps prevent thyroid diseases. Since iodine is often under-supplied in the diet, getting it in the salt you buy helps ensure your family is getting enough. However, some think—because iodine is now so prevalent in salt—we may be getting too much. Kosher salt is another good alternative. It does not contain any additives, including iodine.

Nuts

GENERAL CONCERNS Nuts should not be eaten after the oils have gone rancid. Make sure nuts are fresh; avoid any that are discolored, shriveled, or rubbery, any that look moldy, or any that taste stale. If you buy nuts in bulk, ask the store for permission to taste a sample before buying in quantity.

Be vigilant about peanuts and peanut butter, because carcinogenic aflatoxin can grow on moldy nuts. Others vulnerable to aflatoxin are almonds, Brazil nuts, pecans, pistachios, and walnuts. If you grind nut butter in the store, make sure the machine is thoroughly cleaned.

Whole nuts store best; when nuts are sliced or broken, they can become rancid more quickly. "Slivered" almonds are particularly vulnerable.
BEST CHOICE 100 percent nuts.
ALERT Corn oil (the container is coated in oil), artificial coloring (in red pistachios), salt.

Roasted Nuts

BEST CHOICE 100 percent nuts.
ALERT Hydrogenated oils, flavor enhancers, salt, thickening agents.

Dry-Roasted Nuts

BEST CHOICE 100 percent nuts.
ALERT Salt, corn syrup, flavor enhancers. Other than plain nuts,

these are the most healthful, without added oil and salt.

Nut Butters

BEST CHOICE Freshly ground nuts, such as peanuts.
ALERT Partially hydrogenated oils, corn syrup, sugar, dextrose, stabilizers, salt. For freshness, buy nut butters in a store that will grind them on the spot. Make sure the machine is cleaned daily, however, to avoid aflatoxin.

Starchy Foods

Pasta

BEST CHOICE Unrefined durum semolina; brown rice; kamut; corn.
CONCERNS You have to look hard to find whole-grain pasta; most has been refined and enriched.

Bread Crumbs

BEST CHOICE Whole-grain flours, leavening, salt, spices.

Jeweled Basmati Rice

This dish conjures up visions of Persian opulence. It was once the food of Persian kings and queens. We've boosted the nutrition of the traditional recipe by using brown basmati rice and by excluding the butter customarily used for a bottom crust. SERVES 8 TO 10

- 3 cups brown basmati rice
- 6 cups vegetable broth or water
- ¾ cup fennel bulb (or celery), diced—reserve fronds for garnish
- ½ cup dried cherries, plus extra for garnish
- ½ cup dried apricots, coarsely chopped, plus extra for garnish
- ½ cup pomegranate seeds (chopped grapes are an easy substitute), plus extra for garnish
- ½ cup shelled pistachios, coarsely chopped, plus extra for garnish
- ½ teaspoon fresh minced ginger
- ¼ teaspoon cardamom
- Salt to taste

1. Rinse rice, and then place it with broth or water in a large pot with a tight-fitting lid.

2. Bring to a boil, stir once, reduce heat, cover and simmer 50 minutes.

3. Leaving the lid on, remove from heat and allow to sit, covered, for 10 minutes.

4. Stir in all other ingredients, reserving extras for garnish.

5. Let cool to room temperature, and serve heaped on a platter garnished liberally with fennel fronds, dried fruit, pomegranate seeds, and nuts.

Cooking & Eating

FLAVOR MAVENS

Learning to base your cooking on flavor and what is fresh, whole, and available locally inspires flexibility and creativity. *The Flavor Bible: The Essential Guide to Culinary Creativity*, by Karen Page and Andrew Dornenburg, is of great help in finding flavorful combinations to go with hundreds of different ingredients. Got Brussels sprouts? The chefs will give you just the right flavor affinities, as well as techniques for cooking.

ALERT Dough conditioners, flavor enhancers, preservatives, partially hydrogenated oils.

OTHER CONCERNS High fat content.

Shake-in-a-Bag Breading Mix

BEST CHOICE Herbs and spices.

ALERT Hydrogenated oils, flavor enhancers, preservatives.

Prepared Meat Glazes

BEST CHOICE None.

ALERT Flavor enhancers, thickening agents, sugar, corn syrup.

Instant Potatoes

BEST CHOICE None.

Rice (Brown, Enriched, Converted, White)

BEST CHOICE Whole brown rice—long-, medium-, or short-grain.

CONCERNS Read the labels of seasoned rice carefully to see if the products contain flavor enhancers, preservatives, and stabilizers.

OTHER CONCERNS When rice is polished and milled to create white rice, many nutrients are lost.

- Instant rice is the least nutritious.
- Enriched rice returns some, but not all, of the nutrients.
- Converted rice, sometimes called parboiled, is the most nutritious of the processed rices. It is steamed and pressurized before milling, forcing 70 percent of the nutrients of the bran and germ into the grain; fiber is unaffected.

Stuffing Mix

BEST CHOICE Whole-grain flour, natural leavening, spices, butter.

ALERT High salt and fat content; flavor enhancers, dough conditioners, preservatives, partially hydrogenated oils.

Cold Cuts

This category includes bologna, corned beef, ham, liverwurst, pastrami, pepperoni, salami, and processed chicken, turkey, and roast beef.

BEST CHOICE Nitrate-free whole turkey or chicken breast cooked and sliced.

ALERT BHT, BHA, other preservatives, nitrates, excessive salt, fat.

Hot Dogs

BEST CHOICE "Uncured turkey frankfurter"; or skip meat altogether by choosing soy/tofu dogs.

ALERT Even chicken frankfurters labeled "healthy" and "low-fat" may contain corn syrup and nitrites.

Snacks

GENERAL GUIDELINES Snacks are notoriously high in fat and sugar. Try to reduce the consumption of "junk food" by substituting whole-food snacks.

Candy

BEST CHOICE (actually best compromise): Maple sugar candy; candy made with natural, not synthetic, dyes.

ALERT Artificial colors, hydrogenated oils, aspartame (NutraSweet or Equal).

Dried Fruit

BEST CHOICE 100 percent dried fruit.

ALERT Sulfiting agents.

- Some fruit may have added sugar.
- Banana chips may be fried.

Chips

BEST CHOICE Potato or corn chips.

ALERT The more flavored the chip, the more likely it contains a number of chemical additives, such as partially hydrogenated oils, artificial flavors, dyes, monosodium glutamate.

OTHER CONCERNS Choose reduced-fat, salt-free, baked (not fried) chips.

"Fruit" Snacks

BEST CHOICE Fruit, water, lemon juice.

ALERT Artificial colors and flavors, sulfites, mineral oil.

OTHER CONCERNS Often packaged with the phrase "snacks made with fruit," these products are sold in the breakfast section. Many have little fruit and quantities of artificial colors and flavors.

Puddings and Gelatin Desserts

BEST CHOICE Real flavor and color; puddings made with whole grains.

ALERT Artificial flavors and colors, preservatives.

Trail Mix

BEST CHOICE Nuts, seeds, unsulfured dried fruit.

ALERT Sulfiting agents.

Soy Products

GENERAL CONCERNS Soy is naturally rich in isoflavones yet is considered to be naturally estrogenic, a fact that is creating controversy about how healthy a food it is. Some feel it protects against diseases, such as breast cancer, and others say that it promotes them.

ALERT Soy cheeses can contain casein, a milk derivative. (This can be of concern to someone who is eating soy cheese in an effort to avoid dairy products due to allergy.)

Soy Milk

BEST CHOICE Manufacturers now fortify soy milks with calcium and vitamin D to make a nutritionally comparable alternative to fortified milk.

ALERT Some soy milks have high fat

Cooking & Eating

KNOW YOUR RICE

The world of rice is a many-hued and many-splendored thing. It is also a highly processed one. In the past, most of the rice sold in the U.S. for direct consumption has been white rice, milled to remove the bran, some of the endosperm, and the germ—which means removing the bulk of rice's protein, fiber, calcium, and minerals.

Brown rice comes in short-, medium-, and long-grain varieties. Long-grain rice cooks up light and fluffy; medium- and short-grain are stickier. Short-grain rice has a slight nutritional edge.

You can buy instant or quick brown rice, which has been subjected to high heat to allow for a quicker cooking time. The nutritional loss isn't huge, but the taste and texture suffer.

If you want to spice up your rice life, look for two unusual and exotic heirloom rice varieties—black and red rice.

Black rice is a short-grained, fragrant rice, high in fiber, with a deep, nutty taste. It turns a rich purple when cooked, primarily because of its high anthocyanin content. It has a high mineral content, including iron.

Bhutanese red rice grows at a high elevation in the ranges of the Himalaya. The minerals in this medium-grain heirloom give it a red color and nutty flavor. Since it is semi-milled, it cooks somewhat faster than an unmilled brown rice does—so, although slightly more refined than non-instant brown rice, it is a good choice when you are short on time.

content, but because they are made from soybeans, most of the fat is unsaturated. Most soy milk companies are producing lower-fat varieties of their soy milk, and a few are unsweetened.

Tofu

BEST CHOICE Tofu; tofu with herbs. You can choose tofu textured "firm," "silken," or "soft."

ALERT Since tofu is highly perishable, it is very important that the tofu you buy is fresh. Unhealthful microorganisms grow on souring tofu. Tofu that is "off" has a sour taste, a slimy feel, and can have a slight discoloration. It should be discarded.

Wash tofu every day and cover it with fresh water. Studies have shown that tofu sold in sealed packages has the lowest bacteria count.

OTHER CONCERNS If you buy tofu in bulk, be sure that it is:

- Covered with filtered water or spring water.
- Kept in a cooler and handled by store employees only. If the tofu is in a deli section, it should not be in the deli case, since most deli cases are kept at 50°F and tofu is best at no higher than 41°F.

Cooking & Eating

POP ART

What fun to know that popcorn is a whole grain! Microwave popcorn should be avoided, though, because of the chemical coating used in the bags and the excess sodium and other unnecessary ingredients added. To make popcorn on your stovetop:

1. Pour 3 tablespoons of olive oil (or grapeseed oil if you prefer a more neutral taste) into a heavy, 3-quart or larger pan and place on medium high heat.

2. Put two kernels in, and when one has popped, pour in ⅓ cup of popcorn kernels (white or yellow) and cover the pan.

3. When the corn begins to pop, shake the pan constantly; this allows steam to escape from the popping kernels—otherwise the popcorn will lose its crunch.

4. Remove the pan from the heat the second the popping stops, or it will burn. Pour popcorn into a large bowl and season to taste.

Alternative Ways of Finding Whole Foods

It can be exciting to step aside from shopping exclusively in conventional food stores and find food in other ways. In fact, you may discover that the most economical and abundant sources of whole, organic foods year-round are found outside of supermarkets. And there are unexpected rewards in alternative shopping, not the least of which is reconnecting with the natural world, the seasons, and learning how your food is grown.

When food is grown on your land, or by farmers you know, spring becomes the season of tender shoots of asparagus, strawberries, and rhubarb, and the dog days of August are passed by eating freshly picked, succulent cucumbers. The bounty of early fall is marked by an abundance of tomatoes and zucchini, and winter is heralded with hearty soups made from harvested root vegetables.

From a strictly practical point of view, finding food in farmers' markets, food co-ops, and other places listed below can save you money. Many people have found that though buying fresh organic food in supermarkets and health food stores can be prohibitively expensive, obtaining produce through alternative methods can be cheaper.

Alternative ways for acquiring food—such as CSAs and farmers' markets—bring us into close contact with the farmers as well as the seasons. Growers can chat with us about how the growing season is going, while providing food picked that morning.

Not all small-scale farms and orchards, or all CSAs, provide exclusively organic meat, eggs, dairy, fruit, or vegetables. For advice on how to decide among the many options, see When Faced With Choices on page 24.

FARMERS' MARKETS Farmers' markets (also known as green markets) are returning to towns and cities everywhere. In fact, according to the USDA, 17,555 farmers' markets opened in the last decade, whereas 20 years ago there were only 100. Farmers' markets are treasured by farmers and consumers alike. Found deep in the middle of the largest cities, and in smaller towns across America, farmers' markets are usually outdoors, and they are always colorful. Local farmers, bakers, and food-based cottage industries set up in a communal area, once or twice a week or more, to sell their food to the community.

Most farmers' markets sell not only local produce but also local freshly baked goods such as scones, baguettes, focaccia; clotted cream and organic milk in glass bottles from local dairy farms; fiery salsas made from local tomatoes; ranch-raised ducks, chickens, and turkeys; and, of course, produce—basil, cilantro, mesclun, tomatoes, greens, scallions, lettuce of every sort, peppers, apples, pears, and melons. Variety is dependent only on the season. Farmers' markets provide the opportunity for farmers and consumers to meet, and it isn't uncommon for friendships to develop over the course of a season's harvest.

FOOD CO-OPS AND COOPERATIVE-BUYING CLUBS

The National Cooperative Business Association (NCBA) describes food-buying clubs and co-ops as "typically informal groups organized to buy directly from a wholesaler and save substantially on groceries." Group members order in bulk and divide their order among themselves. Each person also volunteers time toward the tasks of ordering, bookkeeping, and distribution. Cooperative buying clubs may be organized to obtain common grocery items or special types of products such as produce, natural foods, or canned goods.

In some states the word "co-op" can apply only to organizations that are legally incorporated. In those states, many co-ops are technically not cooperatives but food-buying clubs that are cooperatively organized. Food co-ops and buying clubs usually need to spend $400 on groceries monthly to pay the discounted prices of a co-op wholesaler. Just two or three households could meet that requirement easily. Most buying clubs work on a preorder and pay-on-delivery system, although some prepay when the order is submitted to the wholesaler.

Start Your Own Food Co-op

To find a local co-op wholesaler or existing buying clubs in your area, a helpful resource is Co-op Directory Services *(www.coopdirectory.org)*. With a small core membership, develop the co-op and establish a vision. Once you have determined the size for your co-op, solicit members through word of mouth, advertising, and the like. Assign key positions: bookkeeper, order compiler, networker for delivery dates or potluck dinners, and those who meet the delivery truck.

Avoid Chemicals and Additives as Possible

Can you imagine eating 150 pounds of additives a year? The average American does; much of it is sugar and salt, but by no means all. Three thousand additives are intentionally used in processed foods. Unintentional additives contribute many thousands of pounds more. What are these additives doing to us?

ARTIFICIAL SWEETENERS Artificial sweeteners include aspartame (brands NutraSweet and Equal), saccharin, and sucralose (Splenda). They have no nutritive value and have not been shown to be successful in weight loss.

The concept of sweetening without adding calories has obvious advantages, but saccharin has been linked to bladder cancer, and the use of aspartame may cause multiple health problems. In the body, aspartame is broken down into amino acids and methanol. Amino acids are naturally occurring compounds that are used in the human body to synthesize proteins. Many researchers

Food can never be perfectly safe, but it can be safe enough when everyone involved—from farmer to consumer—does the right thing.

—**MARION NESTLE, *WHAT TO EAT***

Shopping & Saving

INSPIRATIONAL FOOD CO-OPS

Two cooperative buying clubs have been big parts of my life. Different as night and day, they illustrate the possibilities.

The Hanover Food Cooperative began in the 1940s in Hanover, New Hampshire. It first operated in a garage. Still a cooperative today, it runs not only a large co-op grocery store but also a credit union and a service station.

Another successful food co-op in my life, Green Squash, is low-key in comparison.

A preorder food-buying co-op, it consists of ten families who have little extra time but spare a night a month for a potluck dinner; they also collate orders, do bookkeeping, and divide up deliveries. All of the members save on their food bills. *—A.B.B.*

use the fact that amino acids are "natural" to support their view that aspartame is safe.

SULFITES, SULFUR DIOXIDE GAS There are six sulfites, and the FDA has ranked them as Generally Regarded as Safe (GRAS): sulfur dioxide, sodium sulfite, sodium and potassium bisulfite, and sodium and potassium metabisulfite. The USDA has banned the use of sulfites on meat, since they can give a false impression of freshness by turning it red.

Sulfites can be found in a surprising number of products, including chili, almost all vinegars, dried fruit, potatoes, wine, shrimp, and children's "fruit" snacks. And in some unexpected places: relishes, horseradish, sugar derived from sugar beets (including brown, white, and confectioners'), and some baked goods.

Sulfiting agents can cause death from anaphylactic shock in highly sensitive individuals. The FDA estimates the number of individuals sensitive to sulfites as 1 in 100; 5 percent of those with asthma may have worsening of symptoms when exposed to sulfiting agents. Those sensitive to sulfites can have mild to deadly reactions to them. Most sulfite-sensitive people are asthmatics; a typical reaction is difficulty breathing within a number of minutes of eating food containing sulfites. Sulfites are most commonly used to retain color in products such as fruits and vegetables.

MONOSODIUM GLUTAMATE (MSG) MSG is a sodium salt of glutamic acid, an amino acid, and is, according to the FDA's definition, naturally occurring. MSG is often found in Chinese food, so sensitivity to MSG has been dubbed the Chinese restaurant syndrome. Symptoms include headaches, difficulty breathing, tingling in the hands, arms,

SNAPSHOT **RICK SMITH AND BRUCE LOURIE**

"At this moment in history, the image conjured up by the word 'pollution' is just as properly a rubber duck as it is a giant smokestack."

Toronto, Canada

Co-authors, *Slow Death by Rubber Duck: How the Toxic Chemistry of Everyday Life Affects Our Health*

Two prominent Canadian environmentalists decided to deliberately ingest a whole bunch of everyday suspect substances and see whether they did, in fact, increase chemicals such as bisphenol A (BPA) and mercury in their systems. Their eating habits had to resemble those of everyday life—eating canned food and tuna fish, for example. One outcome: their blood levels of BPA increased 7.5 times after eating canned foods out of a microwavable, polycarbonate plastic container. To learn more alarming details, visit their website: *www.slowdeathbyrubberduck.com.*

and neck, heart palpitations, and numbness. MSG can be a serious threat to some asthmatics.

As with aspartame, when amino acids are thrown out of balance, there can be serious consequences. For example, infant mice fed large amounts of MSG suffered damage to the hypothalamus; the same result has been seen in monkeys.

While maple syrup is quite high on the glycemic index (54), it has the fewest calories per volume of any sweetener other than honey. It is also rich in antioxidants and the minerals manganese, zinc, calcium, and iron.

SODIUM NITRATE AND SODIUM NITRITE Sodium nitrate is used to preserve meat and help it retain its color. It is commonly found in many luncheon meats. Sodium nitrate alone is considered harmless, but it combines with saliva and bacteria to become nitrite, which the body converts into nitrosamines—powerful

Healthy for You

PLEASE PASS ON THE SALT

The average American consumes about three teaspoons of salt a day. Those who eat a lot of convenience, processed, and prepackaged foods are probably getting much more salt than they can imagine.

Read the labels carefully on canned soups, baked goods, dairy products such as cheese, pickles, and other fermented foods. One can of soup can have 750 milligrams of salt; two slices of bread, 250 milligrams; and 3 ounces of ham, a whopping 1,000 milligrams. Watch out for ham, which can have more than 1,000 milligrams of sodium in just 3 ounces. Vegetables frozen or canned with a sauce can contain almost 500 milligrams of sodium in just one half cup.

Look instead for labels marked "low-sodium" (140 milligrams or less per serving), "very low sodium" (35 milligrams or less), or "sodium-free" (less than 5 milligrams), especially when you are buying packaged foods. And, in general, try to reduce your family's consumption of high-sodium products such as dill pickles, bouillon, olives, and soy sauce.

SNAPSHOT **HEIDI SWANSON**

"Think about how your cooking could change if you eliminated all-purpose white flour, white sugar, and other highly processed ingredients."

San Francisco, California

Author, *Super Natural Cooking*
Blogger, *www.101coobook .com*; *www.mighty foods.com*

Heidi Swanson pulls recipes from vintage and out-of-print cookbooks for her blog, *www.101cookbooks.com.* Sometimes she builds off a recipe she finds. Other times she chooses recipes that intersect with events in her life, her travels, and her everyday interests. Ideas might come from her cookbook collection, or they might come from a friend or a family member—and, now and then, she will just up and create a new recipe from scratch.

carcinogens. Vitamins C and E reportedly help inhibit the development of the nitrosamines. While avoidance of meats containing sodium nitrate is the best course, whenever you eat meats that have nitrates in them, eat a pear or orange for vitamin C as well.

Agave is a light, sweet syrup that comes from the same plant—the agave—as does tequila. The plant thrives in southern Mexico and was prized by the Aztecs. Agave, very low on the glycemic index, is a gift to those with metabolic syndrome, insulin resistance, or diabetes.

ARTIFICIAL FOOD COLORING The Center for Science in the Public Interest charges that food colorings are linked to hyperactivity and behavior problems in children and should be prohibited from use in foods. The group has petitioned the FDA to ban these eight food colors on the market in the U.S: Yellow 5, Red 40, Blue 1, Blue 2, Green 3, Orange B, Red 3, and Yellow 6. Many of these dyes are already being phased out in the United Kingdom.

The FDA has estimated that between 47,000 and 94,000 Americans are sensitive to Yellow 5. It can cause asthma, hives, headache, and is linked to behavioral changes. In a double-blind study reported in the *Journal of Pediatrics,* children were tested to see if Yellow 5 could trigger behavioral reactions. The study clearly demonstrated a relation between the ingestion of Yellow 5 and behavior changes in children allergic to it.

BHT AND BHA Butylated hydroxytoluene (BHT) and butylated hydroxyanisole (BHA) are commonly used to reduce rancidity in foods such as cereals and crackers. The World Health Organization lists BHA as a possible carcinogen and an endocrine disrupter. BHT—prohibited in England—may be toxic to the kidneys and may have a deleterious effect on those who take steroid hormones and oral contraceptives. It is sometimes used to treat packaging. If BHT and BHA are added to an ingredient used in a processed food, they need not be specifically listed. To avoid them, avoid processed foods.

Quinoa Risotto

Technically this isn't risotto—which would imply a dish made from rice. But calling it "quinotto" might be a little too cute. Substitute the protein superstar quinoa for the refined Arborio rice used in risotto. This is a basic recipe—at the end of cooking, add mushrooms, carrots, greens, or whatever veggies you fancy. **SERVES 6**

- 1 tablespoon olive oil
- 2 chopped shallots
- 1 minced garlic clove
- 1 cup quinoa, well rinsed
- 2 cups vegetable stock
- ¼ cup grated Parmesan cheese
- Salt and pepper to taste

1. In a large saucepan, saute the shallots and garlic in olive oil until the shallots become translucent.

2. Add the quinoa and cook for about one minute, stirring.

3. Add 1 cup of the stock and stir until absorbed. Continue adding stock by the half cup until it is all absorbed and the quinoa is cooked. It should be tender, but still have a bit of texture.

4. Stir in the cheese and season with the salt and pepper.

Shoestring Zucchini with Rosemary

Zucchinis are the rabbits of the vegetable world: Turn around, and there's a whole new batch right before your very eyes. Here is a recipe to make good use of all those squashes. SERVES 2 TO 4

- 1 very large zucchini
- 1 teaspoon salt
- ½ cup olive oil
- 2 tablespoons white whole wheat flour (or unbleached all-purpose)
- Several sprigs of rosemary

1. Cut the squash lengthwise into halves, and then cut into ¼-inch slices, then cut those into ⅛-inch slices.

2. Sprinkle and toss with salt in a colander and set in the sink to drain for 30 minutes. After draining, squeeze out as much water as you can with your hands.

3. Heat oil in a skillet—you want the oil very hot, but not smoking.

4. Toss zucchini with flour in a bowl, then add it to the oil in batches. Cook for about 5 minutes until zucchini is just golden, then toss in a few leaves of rosemary. Cook for another minute until zucchini is golden.

5. Drain zucchini on paper towel and serve immediately.

Healthy for You

TAKE THE SHAKER TEST

The daily allowance of sodium, or table salt, recommended for an adult by the National Academy of Sciences is only 500 milligrams a day—less than a quarter of a teaspoon! To find out how much salt you actually add to your food, take the shaker test recommended by the USDA.

Serve yourself a normal dinner plate. Cover it with wax paper, and salt your meal as you would normally. Collect the salt in the wax paper and measure it.

STEP 7

Stock Your Pantry

The modern pantry has expanded beyond the first French *paneterie*—storeroom for bread—to a place for storing dry and canned foods. Today it is more than just a shelf or a cupboard. In fact, it might be a whole room. Make yours a green pantry, purged of unhealthy items and stocked with nourishing staples. Transform it from a storeroom into a culinary adventure.

WHAT IT MEANS

A Green Pantry

Replace refined foods with whole-food staples, so you are always ready to cook and serve true food.

Keeping a green pantry is a simple concept: Weed out the junk food, processed items, and refined staples, and replace them with healthy snacks, natural items, and whole staples. As a species, we've survived and evolved just fine without relying on industrial food. Indeed, the history of how grains, nuts, dried beans, and herbs and spices fanned out across the world is fascinating, involving the travels of explorers and the meanderings of the spice and silk trades. Soybeans and adzuki beans came from China, lentils from the Mediterranean; black-eyed peas gained popularity in Africa after being imported from China; chickpeas came from India; and black, pinto, and red kidney beans came from the Americas. Cookbooks of the world's foods are gold mines of information about interesting and flavorful ways of using this world of staples.

WHY IT MATTERS FOR YOU

A Requisite Tool

Stock up on staples so that cooking healthy meals is always convenient as well as nutritious.

A pantry full of whole grains and flours, nuts and seeds, dried beans and peas, teas and oils, is a tool for making cooking with whole foods convenient. These foods are also excellent sources of nutrition, providing fiber, complex carbohydrates, essential fatty acids, crucial minerals such as zinc and iron, and more. The nutritional benefits of these foods cannot be emphasized enough. All you need to add for a well-balanced diet are fresh fruits and vegetables, and dairy and other animal products if you choose. Pantry foods are versatile and can be used to make delicious, flavorful meals.

WHY IT MATTERS FOR EARTH

Less Ecological Harm

A plentiful, green pantry means fewer packaged foods and less trash.

The most important step in this book is the one that doesn't get a chapter: eating home-cooked meals made from nutritious ingredients. It's better for your health, your wallet, and the planet. The secret to delicious home cooking is a well-stocked pantry with the basic building blocks for any meal. A pantry stocked with Earth's bounty is low on packaged foods, low on heat-and-eat fast foods, and low on foods laden with added sugars, salts, and preservatives. It's filled with whole-grain flours for making delicious waffles and breads, fresh syrup and honey for spreading on top, nut butters and local jams for snacks, and a variety of oils, dried fruits, herbs, and spices for adding flavor to dishes. A pantry should be your store of Earth's delights, all produced with the least ecological harm, none processed in ways that reduce nutritional value.

A well-stocked pantry is also the best way to significantly reduce the packaging your household sends out to the trash. Having a good pantry means buying in bulk, reusing glass jars for storage, and thinking in terms of supplies. This shift in concept—working and planning meals from the perspective of supplies instead of products—has a profound effect on how we shop.

Instead of flour thickener, use 1 tablespoon arrowroot to 2 ½ tablespoons all-purpose flour.

HOW TO DO IT

Fast or Slow

Take your choice: the quick purge or the slow swap. Either method means a step forward.

Presuming that your pantry needs a serious overhaul, you can either go through every item and remove those that are refined, not whole, or those that contain artificial ingredients. (Compost them, use them for pet food, donate them.) Or you can wait until you run out of an item and then replace it with its healthier cousin, one at a time.

Learning from our ancestors: Ancient grains such as quinoa are gaining widespread popularity due to their high protein and nutrient content and appealing taste.

Grains and Flours

Cereal grains are the fruits of the grass family. Wheat, rye, barley, oats, corn, millet, and rice are all true cereals. (Some seeds and berries—buckwheat, for example—are also treated as grains although they are not in fact from the grass family.) A typical grain kernel is made up of a hull or husk, which protects the whole; bran, which holds the kernel together; the germ or embryo, which is the grain's seed and contains about 90 percent of the nutritional content of the kernel; and the endosperm, which is mostly starch. Grain kernels are steel-cut, rolled, flaked, or ground into meals and flours.

Whole grains are important sources of complex carbohydrates, starch, and fiber. Oats and many other grains contain components that help the body reduce high serum cholesterol levels, and fiber that helps reduce insulin elevations after eating. Whole grains are a main staple in diets all over the world.

Most flours are derived from a whole cereal grain milled into a fine meal; the flour is then used for making baked goods. Modern milling puts the whole cereal grain through a high-heat process that removes the germ and bran, leaving only the endosperm—the starch—which is then ground into different sizes for different purposes. The result is a "refined" flour. Refined wheat flour is often bleached with chlorine dioxide to make it white, and chemically aged with potassium bromate or iodate to improve its baking properties. Then it is "enriched" by adding some (not all) of the vitamins stripped from the grain during milling.

The stone-ground milling process is the most popular method of milling that does not remove the bran or germ; the result is a whole-grain flour. Mills that produce stone-ground grains exist all across the United States; some are old and still powered by water, others new and powered by electricity. Flours from mills that stone grind are commonly available in health food stores, specialty mail-order catalogs, and green supermarkets. Stone-ground flours are usually identified as such.

To substitute for all-purpose wheat flour, use 3/4 the amount of barley flour.

Cooking & Eating

EASY WAYS TO COOK GRAINS

A good electric grain steamer (commonly called a rice steamer) is a useful tool for cooking whole grains. You can make a whole-grain porridge for breakfast, or flavorful side dishes, cold salads, and additions to soups and stews. Follow manufacturers' directions for steaming times.

In general, use one-quarter to one-half cup less liquid for electric steamers than is called for in stovetop cooking.

(For more on steaming and recommended equipment, see pages 25-29.)

To cook whole grains in a regular pot on a stove, bring the required amount of water to a boil, stir in the grain, return the water to a boil, cover, lower the heat, and cook until the liquid is absorbed. If the grain is not tender, or the liquid is not absorbed, replace the cover and cook a few minutes longer.

Replacing refined grains with whole grains does not mean heavy food. Softer whole grains such as barley, oat, millet, teff, and brown rice grind into flours that are light in texture and color and rich in mellow flavors. Or you can try white whole-wheat flour, a mild, whole-grain alternative. There are many delicious grains and flours, both familiar and unfamiliar: barley, buckwheat, kamut, oats, quinoa, rice, spelt, teff, and triticale.

Barley needs to be cooked for a while to become chewy. Soak the grain overnight to reduce cooking time. Cook until chewy.

FRESHNESS AND STORAGE Millers of the early 20th century were delighted with the new, high-heat milling process that removed both bran and germ; the germ no longer gummed up the grinding mill, and removal of the oil greatly extended the flour's shelf life. But the germ oil is rich in vitamin E, so whole-grain flour is the most nutritious. Unlike refined flour, it does not have a long shelf life, however, because the living oil in the germ becomes rancid over time. Whole-grain flours should be either ground right before use (the ideal solution) or bought in small quantities and stored in the refrigerator or freezer—like perishable fruits and vegetables—until use, no longer than a month. Even refined flours should be kept no more than six months.

Small, manual flour mills are available for around $60. Small electric flour mills that grind with stone cost around $250. Grinding your own flours does not take much effort and will provide you with high-quality flours rich in flavor and nutrition.

Unhulled grains can last for centuries. The hull completely protects the oils from rancidity. Before cooking, grains in their hull need to be soaked to soften the hull, which will speed along the cooking. Always rinse grains thoroughly before using.

Simple Stewardship

PANTRY PESTS

A pantry full of grains is lovely; a pantry filled with grain moths—not so nice. When you bring food into your house, chances are that some insect pests might come along. The peskiest of pests stow away for a free ride into your pantry, often in sealed packages straight from the store. The pests most often encountered in stored food products are Indian meal moths; dermestid beetles; sawtoothed grain beetles; cigarette and drugstore beetles; flour beetles; granary, rice, and maize weevils; bean weevils; and spider beetles.

Of these, the Indian meal moth is the most common and troublesome pantry pest. Often mistaken for clothes moths, you may find the larvae in food packages along with webbing, cast skins, and frass—the debris left behind after insects have been eating. You will also see the adult moths flying around your kitchen and home.

To Control Indian Meal Moths

- When purchasing milled grain products, flour, and dried fruit, look for broken and damaged packages and boxes—as well as infestation—to avoid bringing stored pests accidentally into your home.
- Cut down on storage time of susceptible foods by purchasing seldom-used foods in small quantities. Decant milled grain products into insect-proof containers of glass or metal with screw-top lids; plastic bags are worthless (pests burrow right in). Store susceptible foods in fridge or freezer.
- At the first sign of infestation, find the source and quickly get rid of it. Dispose of heavily infested foods or bury in your garden. If detection is made early, you can solve the problem easily.
- Careful cabinet cleaning is the best method to avoid stored product pests. Remove every thing from the storage area; vacuum shelves, especially cracks and crevices. Scrub surfaces with soap and hot water.
- Place bay leaves in the storage bins, boxes, or jars—grains do not absorb the flavor, and the leaves keep moths "at bay."

Guide to Whole Grains and Flour

Amaranth

About the size of a poppy seed, this small seed with an unusually high amino acid content was a staple of ancient Native Americans. Not actually a grain, but an excellent protein. Contains no gluten.

Whole Amaranth

USES Breakfast cereal (boiled), popped (like popcorn), side dishes like rice or salads. Sticky and glutinous; use in a 1:3 ratio with other grains.

Amaranth Flour

Substitute equally up to ¼ cup.

Arrowroot

The starch of the maranta root, used as a grain substitute. No gluten.

Ground/powdered Arrowroot

USES A thickener; substitute equally for cornstarch.

Barley

A cereal grain with a nutty flavor. Low amounts of gluten.

Whole Barley

The most nutritious barley, with only the husk removed.

USES Salads, breads, baked goods, pilafs, hot cereals. Soak grain overnight to reduce cooking time.

Barley Flour

Light, resembling refined white flour. Contains little gluten, so combine with higher gluten flour for yeast breads.

USES Quick breads, muffins, and scones.

Pearl Barley

A more refined barley.

USES Soups, casseroles, salads. Steam with broth for casseroles, salads; simmer in soup one hour.

Barley Flakes

Made from pearl barley.

USES Hot cereal or added to breads. For cereal, cook equal parts barley flakes and water.

Buckwheat/Kasha

A seed, not in wheat family, containing all eight amino acids. Roasted buckwheat groats are commonly called kasha. Small amount of gluten.

Whole Buckwheat

USES Pilafs, breads; use like rice.

Buckwheat Flour

Dark flour, from roasted buckwheat.

USES Pancakes and muffins.

Soba Noodles

Japanese noodles made of roasted buckwheat and wheat.

Udon Noodles

Japanese noodles made of unroasted buckwheat and wheat.

Chickpea Flour/Besan Flour

High-protein flour made from ground, unroasted chickpeas. No gluten.
USES Falafel, Indian fritters; thickener.

Corn/Maize

Served in many ways—from cornbread to corn on the cob to popcorn—corn ranges in color from yellow to rust to blue-black. Does not contain gluten.

Cornmeal

Mix half and half with refined wheat flour for cornbread.
USES Quick breads; experiment by substituting cornmeal, brown rice, barley, or millet flour for refined flour.

Blue Cornmeal

USES Same as cornmeal; excellent for tortillas.

Polenta

A finely ground Italian cornmeal, polenta resembles cream of wheat.
USES Serve as a side dish.

Hominy

A round kernel, with hull removed and kernel dried.
USES Add to casseroles and bake. Soak in water or milk for 8 hours and cook at low heat for 3-5 hours.

Grits

Ground hominy.
USES Side dish. Cook to consistency of mushy hot cereal.

Masa Harina

Also a form of ground hominy.
USES Tortillas and corn chips

Popcorn

Heat whole corn kernels in covered pan until they explode into fluffy balls about five times their size.

Corn Pastas

100 percent corn noodles are available in most health food stores.

Kamut

Traced to 4000 B.C., this cereal grain with a rich, buttery flavor is making a comeback. Does not contain gluten.

Whole Kamut

Whole kamut will cook faster if soaked for many hours.
USES Hot cereal, side dish, salad.

Kamut Flour

Lighter than whole wheat.
USES Muffins, breads, all wheat-based recipes.

Kamut Flakes

USES Like oatmeal.

Kamut Pastas

Available in health food stores.

Millet

A true cereal grain, related to sorghum. Does not contain gluten.

Whole Millet
USES Soups and stews, breakfast cereals, side dish.

Millet Flour
USES Quick breads such as muffins.

Millet Flakes
USES Like oatmeal.

Oats

A true cereal grain. Contains gluten.

Oat Groats
Oat kernel, hull removed but germ and bran intact.
USES Side dish, pilaf.

Cut Groats
USES Hot cereal; baked goods, such as breads and cookies.

Rolled Oats
Cut groats, steamed to soften, and then rolled into flakes.
USES Same as cut groats.

Quick Oats
Like rolled oats, cut finer; less flavorful than quick oats.
USES Hot cereal for a fast breakfast.

Instant Oats
Finest cut of the oat; resulting hot cereal is mushy and less flavorful.
USES Hot cereal for a faster breakfast.

Oat Bran
Not a whole food; germ and endosperm are removed from oat kernel.

Potato Flour

The starch from potatoes. No gluten.
USES Thickener; flour substitute in gluten-free diets. A flavorless powder, it can be substituted equally for cornstarch for thickening; for a baked dish, substitute ⅝ cup potato flour for 1 cup white flour.

Quinoa

Related to buckwheat and amaranth, quinoa is a tiny complete-protein seed that cooks quickly; sometimes called "vegetarian caviar." It does not contain gluten.

Whole Quinoa
USES Hot cereal, salads, side dishes, served like rice.

Rice

An aquatic cereal grain, rice is a staple around the world. No gluten.
USES Casseroles, side dishes, salad.

Arborio
USES Risotto; available in white and brown varieties.

Basmati
Aromatic rice traditionally grown in Pakistan and India and aged for one year; also grown in the U.S.

Brown Rice
Least processed form of rice; outer hull removed, but not the bran.

Della
An aromatic rice similar to basmati.

Jasmine
Aromatic; stickier than basmati and della rice.

Long-, Medium-, Short-Grain
Refers to length in relationship to width: Long-grain rice is 4–5 times longer than wide.

Parboiled or Converted Rice
Soaked, steamed, and dried before milling; more nutritious than white rice.

Rice Bran
The bran and germ of the rice grain; not a whole food.
USES Added to cereals and baked goods.

Green Pantry Granola

Homemade granola is easy to make and much cheaper than store-bought. It can be made exclusively with supplies in your green pantry. It's also a terrific recipe for getting kids involved. Start with a giant mixing bowl. Let them help determine which ingredients to add—and let them toss and stir. The following recipe is just a general guideline; mix and match to your (healthy) heart's content. MAKES APPROXIMATELY 5 CUPS

- 2 cups rolled oats
- ½ cup applesauce
- ¼ cup maple syrup
- 2 tablespoons honey
- ¼ cup Sucanat
- 1 cup whole nuts (almonds, walnuts, cashews, pecans, etc.)
- ½ cup large seeds (sunflower seeds, hemp seeds, pepitas)
- ¼ cup sesame seeds
- 1 teaspoon sea salt
- 1 teaspoon ground cinnamon
- ½ teaspoon ground ginger
- 1 tablespoon oil
- 2 cups dried fruit (tart cherries, for example)

1. Preheat oven to 325°F. In a large mixing bowl, mix everything together except the fruit.

2. Spread the mixture out on 1 large or 2 medium baking sheets with rims and place in oven.

3. Several times during baking, stir the mix around with a spatula to ensure even baking.

4. Bake until granola is evenly golden, about 40 to 60 minutes, depending on your oven.

5. Let cool, stir in fruit, and store in airtight bags or containers.

Rice Flour
Look for brown rice flour—it's very delicate and light.
USES Baked goods, such as muffins.

Texamati
Similar to basmati, it is a crossbreed of basmati and long-grain rice. Grown in Texas, it is available as brown rice or refined white.

Wehani
A basmati hybrid with a reddish color.

White Rice
Also referred to as "polished," the hull, bran, and most of germ is removed in the milling process (refined).

Rye

A strong-flavored cereal, often mixed with wheat in breads. Low gluten.
USES Bread; side dishes such as pilaf.

Rye Berries
USES Side dishes, casseroles, salad.

Rye Flour
The darker the flour, the more bran retained during milling. Pumpernickel is the least refined of rye flours.

Cracked Rye
Coarse meal.

Rye Flakes
Cereal like oatmeal.

Sorghum

Related to millet. No gluten.

Whole Sorghum
USES Like rice or millet; used in Africa for flat unleavened bread.

Soy Flour

High-protein soybean flour. No gluten.
USES Substitute up to ¼ cup soy flour for ¼ cup white flour.

Spelt

Related to wheat but has not been hybridized. Contains gluten.

Spelt Berries
USES Side dish, like rice.

Spelt Flakes
USES Like oatmeal.

Spelt Flour
USES Substitute for wheat equally.

Tapioca

Starch from a tropical root; a grain substitute with no gluten.

Pearl Tapioca
USES Tapioca pudding.

Tapioca Flour
USES Substitute for cornstarch or arrowroot for thickening.

Teff

A tiny red, brown, or white seed; white teff is mildest. Contains no gluten.

Whole Teff
USES Hot cereal, alternative to rice.

Healthy for You

ALTERNATIVES TO WHITE PASTA

Most pastas are made from semolina, a refined durum wheat. Only pasta labeled "whole durum wheat semolina" is made of whole grain. For variety, flavor, and breadth of nutrients, try these.

BROWN RICE NOODLES Light-flavored and slightly nutty tasting, rice noodles are fine-textured and virtually identical to "normal" spaghetti.

QUINOA PASTA Quinoa flour is blended with corn or wheat flour to produce a mild-tasting, high-protein pasta. Sensitive to gluten? Look for brands that contain only quinoa and corn flours.

WHOLE WHEAT PASTA Made of 100 percent durum wheat typically, these noodles are higher in fiber, protein, B vitamins, and minerals than semolina varieties, which use only part of the grain. Whole wheat pasta has a hearty flavor and is a good match with pesto and other flavorful sauces.

BUCKWHEAT NOODLES Buckwheat flour is an Asian staple that has been used for centuries to make pasta. Japanese soba noodles are the most common type in the U.S., mildly flavored and high in protein and dietary fiber.

TOFU SHIRATAKI These interesting noodles are made from a mix of soy protein and yam flour. They come packaged in water and are low on the glycemic index and high in soluble fiber.

Teff Flour

USES Commonly made into Ethiopian injera bread, teff flour is mild and light.

Triticale

A hybrid cereal grain—cross between wheat and rye—triticale is more nutritious than either. Contains gluten.

Triticale Berries

USES Breakfast cereal, side dishes.

Triticale Flakes

USES Like oatmeal.

Triticale Flour

USES Substitute equally for wheat or rye flour.

Wheat

The primary grain in the American diet, processed to many stages of refinement. Wheat contains gluten.

Wheat Berries
The entire wheat kernel—germ, endosperm, and bran—except for hull.

Bulgur
Wheat kernel that is steamed, dried, and ground.

Wheat Flakes
Whole wheat kernels that are cut.

Couscous
Made from durum semolina.

Cracked Wheat
Whole wheat kernels dried and cracked (not cooked) between rollers.

Farina
Finely ground cracked wheat.

Durum
Hard wheat; higher gluten content than soft wheat.

Seitan
Often used as a meat substitute, the bran of seitan is rinsed away, leaving the gluten, which is kneaded into a meatlike texture. High in protein.

Soft Wheat
Low-gluten wheat.

All-Purpose/White Flour
Refined wheat flour, with germ and bran removed in milling. All-purpose flour turns white naturally, but some all-purpose flours are bleached and bromated.

Whole Wheat Flour
Milled to retain the bran and the germ; darker than white flour and more flavorful, with denser texture.

White Whole Wheat Flour
Whole-grain flour made with albino wheat; has the nutrition of whole wheat and milder flavor.

Bread Flour
From high-gluten refined hard wheat.

Graham Flour
A whole-grain flour.

Pastry/Cake Flour
Refined white flour; made from low-gluten soft wheat.

Semolina
Made from durum wheat; bran and germ are removed during milling unless the label says "100 percent unrefined durum semolina."

Wild Rice

A North American aquatic grass seed grain hand-picked in the wild.
USES Add to rice dishes for flavor and texture; expensive.

The study of bread making is of no slight importance, and deserves more attention than it receives.

—**FANNIE FARMER, *THE BOSTON COOKING-SCHOOL COOKBOOK* (1918)**

Dried Beans and Peas

Dried beans are extremely versatile. Herbs and spices can transform them into anything from hummus to black bean soup to Mexican tacos. Beans are not complete proteins (the only exception being the soybean) because they lack one or more of the essential amino acids; yet, according to nutritionists, they become perfect proteins when combined with whole grains, nuts, seeds, or animal products.

Beans are a superb source of protein, complex carbohydrates, and soluble fiber; they have only a small percentage of fat, if any, and no cholesterol. Rich in vitamins and minerals, particularly calcium and iron, beans are great foods for diabetics, hypoglycemics, and those with insulin resistance, because they do not trigger the release of excessive insulin.

Dried beans are legumes, the dried seeds from pods of plants. There are approximately 13,000 species of beans, from 600 genera. While we only discuss only 10 in the following list, more and more species are finding their way into specialty stores. Called "boutique" beans, some are derived from hybrids and others from heirloom seeds (see Step 2). Some of the more unusual of these include anasazi, appaloosa, black runner, black valentine, calypso, cranberry, Florida butter, Jackson wonder, pigeon, rattlesnake, scarlet runner, speckled lima, winged, and wren's egg. Buying or growing unusual beans from heirloom seeds is an excellent way of protecting biodiversity.

Dried beans should be kept in tightly covered containers in a dry place. Cooked beans can be frozen for four to six months, or kept in the refrigerator for four to five days. For best results, freeze beans as a prepared dish.

Guide To Basic Beans

Adzuki

Small and brown with white keel.

½ CUP COOKED 0 g fat; 7 g fiber.

USES Commonly sprouted; excellent for salads and sweet dishes.

Black Beans

Black, kidney-shaped with white keel.

½ CUP COOKED 0 g fat; 7 g fiber.

USES Mexican, South American, Spanish, Cuban dishes; soups, casseroles.

Black-eyed Peas

Cream-colored with oval black keel.
½ CUP COOKED 0 g fat; 6 g fiber.
USES African and Mexican dishes, soups, casseroles, cooked with greens.

Cannellini/Great Northern Beans

Long, thin, and white.
½ CUP COOKED 0 g fat; 6 g fiber.
USES Italian dishes, pastas, salads, soups, stews, Boston baked beans.

Chickpeas/Garbanzos

Round and tan, about ¼ inch wide.
½ CUP COOKED 2 g fat; 5 g fiber.
USES Famous in Middle Eastern dishes: falafel, hummus; good for salads, stews.

Kidney Beans

Maroon and kidney-shaped.
½ CUP COOKED 0 g fat; 6 g fiber
USES Chilis, stews, salads.

Lentils

Round and flat—red, yellow, green, or brown.
½ CUP COOKED 0 g fat; 6-8 g fiber.
USES Dhal, soups, stews, side dishes.

Navy Beans

White, similar to the cannellini bean.
½ CUP COOKED ½ g fat; 8 g fiber.
USES Soups, stews, salads.

Pinto Beans

Tan with brown speckles, ½ inch long.
½ CUP COOKED 0 g fat; 7 g fiber.
USES Chilis, stews, salads, tacos.

Soybeans

Small, round, and tan; black soybeans are used in Chinese black bean sauces.
½ CUP COOKED 8 g fat; 5 g fiber.
USES Bean curd (tofu), stir-fry dishes, salads, stews.

Cooking & Eating

SUBSTITUTING CANNED BEANS FOR FRESH

The flavor of canned beans isn't as fresh and rich as home-soaked and cooked, nor is there as rich a variety available. However, having some canned beans in your pantry for a quick dinner can be convenient. The general rule is that a pound of soaked and cooked beans equals approximately 5 to 6 cups. When substituting, two to three 15- or 16-ounce cans of beans are equivalent to a pound of cooked beans. Each can of beans yields about 1¾ cups.

Cooking & Eating

SOAKING BEANS

As a rule of thumb, use 2 to 3 cups of water for each cup of beans.

SOAKING OVERNIGHT
All dried beans, except lentils and peas, need to be soaked—ideally overnight—to soften before cooking. Before soaking, wash the beans thoroughly. When soaking is complete, rinse the beans thoroughly.

QUICK-SOAK METHOD
If you forget to soak beans overnight, there is an alternative. Soak as long as possible, rinse, and then place in a pot and cover with water. Bring the beans to a rapid boil for 3 to 4 minutes, remove from heat, cover, and let sit for an hour. Wash the beans thoroughly, replenish the water with clean water, and proceed with the recipe. If soaked for a few hours before the quick boil, beans generally need only about half an hour of actual cooking time to reach the right texture and softness.

PRESSURE COOKER METHOD
To save time, use a pressure cooker to cook dried beans. They can be thoroughly cooked in a pressure cooker in about 15 or 20 minutes.

TIPS

- Increase cooking and soaking time in hard water and in high-altitude areas.
- Add ⅛ teaspoon baking soda to the pot if you have hard water.
- Add seasonings in the beginning; add salt only after the beans are tender.
- Acids slow the softening of beans. Add acid-based foods such as tomatoes as late in the cooking process as possible.
- Mexican cooks cook their beans with the herb epazote to reduce flatulence. Coriander, cumin, and ginger reportedly also have that effect.
- Add olive oil to the cooking water to reduce foaming and boiling over.
- Remove beans from heat and let cool in the cooking water to prevent them from drying out.
- When beans and grains are combined, complete proteins are formed with all of the essential amino acids.
- Slow cookers do not simmer at high enough heat to cook beans, although it would seem like such a good idea! In truth, it would take 16 hours or more.

For freshest flavor, buy cardamom seedpods, not ground cardamom, then crush them lightly to get out the small black seeds. Grind them yourself or use them whole.

Dried Herbs and Spices

From zesty marinades to winter minestrone, herbs and spices help bring grains and beans from your pantry to life. With their rich diversity of flavors, herbs and spices complement ethnic dishes from around the world: earthy-flavored black bean enchiladas with chilis; tomato-based pasta with basil and oregano; East African paprika-based stew with lentils. All can be provided from a full pantry; you only have to add seasonal fruits and vegetables.

Greens and Beans "Burger"

These healthy vegan patties include a few perishables; the rest you can pull from your pantry. SERVES 4

- 4 tablespoons ground flaxseeds
- 12 tablespoons hot water (or hot vegetable stock)
- 2 ½ cups canned garbanzos, drained and rinsed (look for brands that use cans free of BPA)
- ½ teaspoon salt
- ½ teaspoon black pepper
- ¾ cup chopped fresh herbs (cilantro, basil, dill, etc), or 2 tablespoons dried herbs
- 1 onion, chopped
- 1 small orange, grated zest only
- 1 cup greens, finely chopped (spinach, dandelion, arugula, etc)
- 1 cup toasted bread crumbs (whole-grain)
- 1 tablespoon olive oil

1. Mix the flaxseeds with hot water or stock; soak for 10 minutes until texture is gelatinous, like rice pudding.

2. Combine garbanzo beans, flaxseed mix, salt, and pepper in a food processor and process until mixture is thick and creamy, but still a little chunky.

3. Pour into a bowl and stir in herbs, onion, zest, and greens. Gently stir in the bread crumbs and let mix sit for a few minutes, until it is easy to handle and can be formed into 1-inch-thick patties. If it feels too dry, add a little water; if too moist, add bread crumbs.

4. To cook on the stove, use a heavy skillet and heat oil over medium heat. Cook patties, covered, for about 7 minutes or until bottoms begin to brown; flip and cook for another 7 minutes.

5. To cook on the grill, rub both sides of patties with olive oil and grill for 4 minutes per side.

Most herbs and spices are now grown in the United States. But though spices such as cardamom have to be imported, even those who believe most staunchly in eating locally agree that the environmental cost of transporting spices is low (because they are light and a minuscule amount is needed). Try to buy U.S.- and locally grown herbs whenever possible.

SPICES Whereas herbs are derived from leaves, spices are dried seeds, pods, roots, and other plant parts that are usually ground to fine powders. A very short list from the amazing world of spices could include allspice, anise pepper (Szechuan pepper), caraway seeds, cardamom seeds, cassia, celery seed, cinnamon, clove, coriander, cumin, dill seed, fennel seed, ginger, lemongrass, mace, mustard seed, nutmeg, pepper, saffron, and turmeric.

Coriander, cumin, and ginger, when used in combination with beans, reportedly diminish flatulence.

Cooking & Eating

CHOOSING AND USING DRIED SEASONINGS

- Whenever possible, buy the whole herb leaf or the whole spice plant part. Once either the leaf or plant part is broken or ground, flavor is lost. Instead, grind spices at home with a mortar and pestle or clean coffee grinder, right before use. Dried herbs also can be crumbled in your hand, or easily broken apart, before using.
- The best time to buy herbs and spices is late fall, shortly after harvest. Store them in a cool, dry, dark cupboard, in airtight containers, or freeze.
- To substitute dried herbs for fresh in a recipe, add three or four times less dried herbs than the recipe calls for.
- Experiment with soaking dried herbs for ten minutes or so before adding to a dish in water that has just boiled or other hot liquid. Heat releases the flavor of the herbs.

Commonly Used Herb and Spice Combinations

BLEND	INGREDIENTS
Bouquet Garni	thyme, parsley, bay leaf, tarragon
Chinese Five-Spice Powder	Szechuan peppercorns, cinnamon, cloves, fennel, star anise, cassia
Cajun Spices	paprika, chili, garlic, allspice, thyme, cayenne
Chili Powder	garlic, oregano, allspice, cloves, cumin seed, coriander seed, cayenne, black pepper, turmeric, mustard seed, paprika
Creole Seasoning	paprika, garlic, thyme, cayenne, oregano
Desserts	cinnamon, cloves, coriander, ginger, nutmeg, mace, cardamom
French	chives, chervil, parsley, thyme, tarragon
Garam Masala / Indian Dishes	cumin, coriander, cardamom, black pepper
Indian Curry	coriander seeds, cumin, nutmeg, cardamom seed, turmeric, white mustard seed, black mustard seed, fenugreek seed, chilis, ginger, peppercorns, garlic, allspice, cinnamon, cayenne, fennel
Italian Blend	oregano, basil, marjoram, tarragon, parsley
Japanese Seven Flavors	anise, pepper, sesame seeds, flaxseeds, rapeseeds, poppy seeds, dried tangerine or orange peel, ground nori seaweed
Mexican Combinations	garlic, cumin, black pepper, cloves, oregano, cilantro, sometimes cinnamon and coriander
Mexican Fajita	ginger, paprika, jalapeño pepper, oregano, mustard, cumin, red pepper, parsley
North and East African Flavors	paprika, cumin, cloves, cardamom, peppercorns, allspice, fenugreek seeds, coriander seeds, ginger, turmeric, cinnamon, cloves
Panch Phoron /Five Indian Spices	cumin, fennel, bay leaf, fenugreek, onion seeds

Guide to Spices and Dried Herbs

Allspice

A member of the pepper family, allspice combines the flavors of clove, cinnamon, nutmeg, and more.
USES Desserts, quick breads, pickling.

Anise

Tastes slightly like licorice.
USES Added to salad, eggs, cheese, stews, and pastries; combines well with cinnamon and bay leaves.

Anise Pepper (Szechuan Pepper)

Not actually a pepper, but very hot.
USES Chinese five-spice powder.

Bay Leaf

Long, thin, two-inch leaf; brittle when dried.
USES Soups, sauces, stews, beans, marinades; combines well with basil, oregano, thyme, garlic.

Caraway Seeds

Small, strong, and nutty-tasting seed.
USES Commonly added to breads, vegetables, eggs, and cheeses.

Cardamom Seeds

Fragrant; sweet with a slightly gingery flavor.
USES Soups, stews, sweet potatoes, pastries; combines well with cumin and coriander.

Cassia

Often called Chinese cinnamon.
USES Chinese five-spice powder.

Celery Seed

A strong celery flavor. Use sparingly.
USES Vegetables, soups, sauces.

Cinnamon

Fragrant with a rich, strong taste.
USES Squashes, apples and other fruit, spice blends native to Asia and the Mediterranean; combines well with nutmeg, ginger, cloves, and cardamom.

Cloves

Pungent and fragrant.
USES Squashes, fruit, spice blends native to Asia and the Mediterranean; combines well with cinnamon, nutmeg, and ginger.

Cumin

Seed with a very strong, rich flavor.
USES Beans, vegetables, curries.

Dill Seed

Strong flavor; does not need any other herbs.
USES Soups, salads, vegetables such as tomatoes and cucumbers, dairy products, crepes, bland foods such as cauliflower, potatoes.

Fennel Seeds

Sometimes confused with anise, as the licorice flavor is similar, but milder.
USES Salads, tomatoes, grains, beans, dairy products.

Fenugreek Seeds

Frequently used in combination with other spices.
USES Curries, African dishes.

Garlic

Pungent, onionlike flavor.
USES Salad dressings, ethnic dishes (Italian in particular).

Ginger

Pungent and flavorful root.
USES Baked goods, desserts, cuisines from Asia and Africa.

Mace

The "jacket" of the nutmeg; milder than nutmeg.
USES Desserts, sauces.

Mustard

Mild (white) to hot (black), mustard has a tangy and spicy flavor; varieties include white, yellow, brown, black.
USES Vinaigrette salad dressings, "mustard," Indian dishes.

Nutmeg

Rich nutty flavor.
USES Desserts such as pumpkin pie, puddings, cakes, cookies.

Pepper

Cayenne
Pungent and fiery hot.
USES Sauces, soups, beans, chilis; combines well with chilis. Cayenne becomes more flavorful when frozen; high in vitamins A and C.

Chili
Hot and spicy.
USES Beans, eggs; chili powder may be a blend of chili, oregano, cumin, and other herbs and spices.

Paprika
Flavorful pepper that is not as hot as cayenne or chilis.
USES European, African, Portuguese, and Spanish recipes.

Peppercorns

Black, white, pink, green—all berries of the same plant, processed differently.
USES Pepper can zing up sweet and savory dishes alike.

Saffron

Fragrant red "threads" are stamens of purple flowering crocus; most expensive spice in the world.
USES Rice; Indian, North African dishes.

Star Anise

Star-shaped seedpod; licorice taste. **USES** Chinese five-spice powder.

Turmeric

Vivid yellow powder with spicy flavor. **USES** Indian dishes, curries.

Vanilla

Long, narrow bean that can be split open and used for flavoring. Choose natural, not artificial, vanilla extract. **USES** Desserts of all kinds.

Cherry Pine Nut Cookies

This is a fun twist on the classic Italian pignoli cookie—gluten-free, with tangy, chewy fruit playing off the sweet and nutty flavors. For a subtle spicy twist, add a few crushed pink peppercorns. MAKES 3½ DOZEN

- 16 ounces almond paste, coarsely crumbled (see note below)
- 1 cup unrefined sugar
- ½ teaspoon salt
- ¾ cup chopped dried cherries
- 2 large egg whites
- 2 tablespoons mild honey
- 1 cup pine nuts

1. Preheat oven to 350°F. Put almond paste in a food processor and pulse until broken up into small bits; add sugar and salt and pulse for one minute or until finely ground.

2. Transfer almond mixture to large bowl and add cherries, egg whites, and honey. Beat with an electric mixer at medium-high speed until smooth and very thick, about 5 minutes.

3. Spoon 1½-inch rounds 1 inch apart onto baking sheets, lined with parchment. Press in pine nuts.

4. Bake cookies until golden, about 12 to 15 minutes. A good trick with these is to switch the baking sheet from the upper to lower third of oven halfway through baking.

5. Slide parchment with cookies onto racks to cool completely, then remove cookies from parchment.

Note: Almond paste can be found in some supermarkets, ordered online, or made from scratch. Grind 1 ½ cups whole blanched almonds in a food processor to a fine powder (about 2 minutes). Transfer to a bowl and mix with 1 cup unrefined sugar. Stir in 2 egg whites, until mixture is smooth. Roll into a log, wrap in parchment paper, and chill for an hour.

Herbal Infusions

A prized herbalist in her community in upstate New York, Fara Shaw Kelsey enlightens tea drinkers about herbal teas to buy and why. If you are confused by the wide array of herbal mixtures available in stores, her advice can help to make sense of them all.

Strictly speaking, tea is made from the leaves of only one plant—*Camellia sinensis*—but we borrow the word to name the brews made from many different herbs. Herbalists also use the term "simples" to describe herbs utilized one species at a time instead of in compound formulas. As Fara Kelsey describes, simples are an excellent starting place. In fact, she advises that you not get involved—either in buying or making your own—in complex tea formulas unless you are knowledgeable about how the herbs are used. Otherwise, you and your family might be drinking stimulating brews before sleep and sleep-inducing potions for breakfast!

Kelsey has nine simples she recommends for every pantry: mint, fennel, dandelion leaf and root, echinacea, nettle, blueberry leaf, gingerroot, and caffeinated green and flowering jasmine teas. Other herbs she likes are oatstraw, red clover, and cardamom.

TO MAKE HERBAL TEA INFUSIONS Take a handful of the dried herb and put it in a glass jar, such as a Mason jar or glass coffeepot. Pour boiling water over it (a stainless steel knife placed in the jar will absorb some of the heat so that the jar doesn't crack) and immediately stir, making sure all the plant material is wet. Quickly cover the jar so that the vapors do not escape. (The vapors contain the plant's volatile oils.) Let the jar sit at room temperature for four hours, or until completely cooled, then refrigerate. Kelsey makes her infusions at night and cools them at room temperature overnight. Before drinking, strain the tea and serve hot or at room temperature.

TRUE TIP

Cool tea bags provide relief when applied to bug bites and minor burns, including sunburn; tannins in tea have anti-inflammatory effects; put a chilled tea bag on puffy eyes.

Feed tea leaves to garden plants—green tea is high in nitrogen—and they will ward off some pests and insects.

Tea has antibacterial properties, which makes leaves great for fighting odors. Sprinkle used tea leaves on carpets and let sit for ten minutes before vacuuming; sprinkle used tea leaves in litter boxes, pet beds, and trash cans.

Guide to Herbal Teas

Blueberry Leaf

Used by the American Indians, blueberry leaf reportedly helps control blood sugar and varicose veins. Richly flavorful, the tea has culinary as well as medicinal uses.

Dandelion Root

Highly nutritious, dandelion root is a diuretic that helps the body remove poisons. It is high in iron, manganese, phosphorous, magnesium, calcium, chromium, cobalt, zinc, and potassium.

Echinacea Root

The American Indians used echinacea root to help heal wounds. Herbalists regard it as a boon to the immune system.

Fennel

Originating in the Mediterranean, fennel is grown in the U.S. Its licorice taste appeals to children. A pleasant dinner tea and natural breath freshener, it is also good for the intestinal tract.

Flowering Jasmine

Originating in China, flowering jasmine also grows in the southern U.S. Flowering jasmine tea includes the flowers and the tea leaves. When water is added, flowers are revitalized and float in the tea—an elegant enhancement for special occasions.

Gingerroot

Slice off a piece of root, pour boiling water over it, let steep for 10 to 15 minutes, and drink with honey. Ginger helps digest fats, aids the circulation, and has a warming effect. A great winter tea.

Green Tea

Buddhist monks extol green tea for health maintenance and longevity. Green tea's tannins contain catechin, said to reduce cancers of the esophagus and stomach and decrease high blood sugar, high blood pressure, and the buildup of "bad" cholesterol (LDL) while having a minimal effect on "good" cholesterol (HDL). It also freshens breath and fights cavities.

Mint

A refreshing tea and soothing nerve tonic, it stimulates digestion. Serve cold on summer days or hot in the winter.

Nettle

Stinging nettle is high in chromium, cobalt, iron, phosphorus, zinc, copper, and sulfur, as well as B-complex vitamins, especially thiamin and riboflavin. Herbalists believe nettle helps restore adrenal and kidney function and stabilizes blood sugar. Nettle is even used in biodynamic compost to facilitate decomposition.

Whole-Food Sweeteners

Making the switch from white sugar to whole-food sweeteners can be difficult, especially when children expect desserts sweetened with white sugar. But desserts made with whole-food sweeteners can be delicious, and even children learn to prefer the more delicate flavors.

Guide to Sweeteners

Agave Nectar (or Syrup)

Obtained from the heart of the agave plant, agave nectar resembles thin honey in colors from pale to dark amber. It dissolves readily in liquids and is sweeter than sugar; the darker the color, the more it tastes like molasses.

Barley and Other Grain Malts

Derived by sprouting, heating, and drying barley, grain malts are the preferred sweetener of macrobiotic eaters, who restrict their diet mostly to grains. Grain malts, close to being a whole food, are neither overly sweet nor highly concentrated.

Coconut Palm Sugar

Made from the nectar of the coconut palm, this sugar has a round, caramel sweetness used not only for desserts but also for curries and savory dishes.

Date Sugar

Made from dehydrated ground dates, date sugar does not dissolve well.

Fruit Juice Concentrates

Made from the juice of apples, grapes, pears, or oranges, reduced in volume and sugars by slow cooking, juice concentrates can be frozen for year-round use.

Granular Fruit Sweeteners

White grape juice and grain sweeteners are dehydrated and granulated.

Honey

A whole food made from flower nectar, honey is "refined" only by the bees. It has few nutrients—but more than refined sugar. Added to tea, honey is good for treating colds and cold symptoms.

NOTE: Honey should *never* be fed to infants.

Jaggery

A barely refined sugar, jaggery is made from sap collected from flower spikes of date palm fronds. The sap is kettle-boiled over an open-hearth fire and the nectar slowly evaporates into a paste; the sugar is then cooled in coconut shell molds. It comes in big chunks and contains iron and beneficial mineral salts.

Maltose

Sprouted grains and cooked rice are heated and fermented until their starches turn to sugar. Maltose is available in Chinese markets.

Maple Sugar

A Native American staple, maple sugar is produced by boiling the water out of maple syrup. The maple flavor is deliciously distinctive and about twice as sweet as refined cane sugar. Both maple syrup and maple sugar are among the least refined sweeteners.

Maple Syrup

It takes 40 gallons of sap from the sugar maple tree to make one gallon of maple syrup. The process involves evaporating the water, yet natural minerals remain. Ounce for ounce, maple syrup has twice as much calcium as milk.

Molasses

Unsulfured molasses comes from the juice of sun-ripened cane; sulfured molasses is a by-product of refined sugar; blackstrap molasses is the residue of the cane syrup after the

Healthy for You

DECEPTIVE SWEETENERS

What are turbinado sugar, raw sugar, and brown sugar?

Turbinado sugar, also called raw sugar, is made in the first pressing of sugarcane. It retains some of the molasses and although it is slightly less refined than regular white sugar, it is still more refined than the wholesome sweeteners we list here. Many people think that brown sugar is a more natural alternative to white sugar; however, most brown sugar is completely refined beet sugar to which cane molasses has been added. Some brown sugars may retain their natural molasses, but most producers use the refined version so that they can carefully control the ratio of molasses to sugar crystals and reduce manufacturing costs.

True Food Sweeteners

What can substitute for ⅓ cup of white or brown sugar?

SWEETENER	EQUIVALENT
Barley, pearl	1 cup cooked
Barley malt	1½ cups
Date sugar	1 cup
Fruit juice concentrate	½ cup
Granular fruit sweeteners	½ cup
Honey	⅓ cup
Maltose	1¼ cups
Maple sugar	1 cup
Maple syrup	½ cup
Molasses	⅓ cup
Rice syrup	1¼ cups
Sorghum syrup	⅓ cup
Unrefined sugar	½ cup

sugar crystals have been separated. Molasses is nutritious: high in calcium, iron, and potassium.

Rice Syrup

Made from rice and sprouted grains, rice syrup is digested slowly and is easier on blood sugar levels than many other sweeteners.

Sorghum Syrup

Sorghum cane juice is boiled down to create sorghum syrup. Naturally resistant to insects, sorghum cane crops require few pesticides.

Stevia

A plant native to the Americas with sweet leaves and buds, stevia is 30 times as sweet as sugar with almost no calories. One to three drops of stevia will sweeten one cup of liquid. Increasingly available, stevia is sold as powder or liquid extract.

Unrefined sugar (Sucanat)

Sucanat is an unrefined sugar product developed by Swiss pediatrician Max-Henri Beguin. Sucanat, like sugar, is made from sugarcane juice with nothing added or taken out except water. Sucanat thus retains the minerals, vitamins, and trace elements from the sugarcane: 1,125 milligrams of potassium (sugar contains 4.5 milligrams) and 1,600 I.U. of vitamin A.

Healthful Oils

Oils are pressed from the seeds and fruit of plants. Unrefined oils are the most nutritious, as they have not been stripped of fat-soluble vitamins A, D, E, and K. They are also the most flavorful, tasting like the nut or seed they have come from. Refined oils, especially those that are mass-marketed, are nutritionally depleted. The essential fatty acids are damaged from the high-heat processing; they are extracted with solvents, refined with chemicals, and contain preservatives. Refined oils also have very little flavor.

Superunsaturated and polyunsaturated unrefined oils such as canola, soy, walnut, and flax oils contain omega-3 and omega-6 essential fatty acids, which are essential to good health. Unrefined oils highest in omega-3 and omega-6 are, in descending order, hemp, flax, pumpkin, canola, walnut, soybean, safflower, sunflower, sesame, rice bran, and almond. Unrefined monounsaturated oils, such as canola, olive, and high-oleic safflower oils, are also important for health and are linked to reducing serum cholesterol. Saturated oils are considered unhealthful oils and are primarily made up of animal fat, although nuts contain some saturated fats. All plant oils are cholesterol-free.

Unfortunately, unrefined oils are fragile and change when heated, smoking and releasing toxic fumes. Refined oils, on the other hand—especially those that are high in monounsaturates—can withstand high heat before breaking down. It is important to have three kinds of oil in

Maple sugar's heady deep flavor is beautifully enhanced by vanilla. Use half a vanilla bean per one cup of maple sugar. Scrape the bean, bury it in the sugar in a recycled jar, and seal tightly. Let it sit for at least one week. Vanilla maple sugar can be used in coffee, on plain yogurt, in baking—wherever sugar is used.

A jazz musician can improvise based on his knowledge of music. He understands how things go together. For a chef, once you have that basis, that's when cuisine is truly exciting.

—CHARLIE TROTTER, CHEF AND RESTAURATEUR

your kitchen: unrefined oils rich in omega-3 and omega-6 to be used in salad dressings and in sauces that are simmered, steeped, and stewed; unrefined olive oil high in monounsaturated fats for medium-heat cooking; and a refined oil high in monounsaturates, such as high-oleic safflower oil, for high-heat cooking.

Unrefined, polyunsaturated, and superunsaturated oils begin to smoke above 375°F. They also have a higher moisture content and fizz at higher temperatures, and important nutrients such as vitamin E are destroyed. Unrefined oils higher in monounsaturated fats such as olive, sesame, corn, peanut, and safflower oils can be heated from 255°F to 350°F.

Only refined oils should be used for temperatures above 350°F. Refined canola, peanut, safflower, sunflower, and walnut oils can be used between 325°F and 400°F. Refined high-oleic safflower and avocado oils are ideal for high-heat cooking of temperatures up to 520°F.

Healthy for You

STORING OILS

Light causes free radicals to develop in oils, oxygen causes rancidity, and heat affects the molecular structure. Store oil in a cool location until the bottle is opened, and once opened, place it in the refrigerator. Unrefined oils go rancid more quickly than refined. Once refrigerated, unrefined oils can last between 5 and 10 months, and refined oils up to 20 months. If you go through some oils very slowly, consider freezing them. In the freezer unrefined oils can last up to 12 months. Rancid oils smell stale and taste bitter.

Five Easy Marinades

The pantry stores some basic ingredients that can create any number of combos. Case in point: marinades. Here are some great mixes that work to transform plain old vegetables into superstars. The alchemy is simple—mix the marinade and let your vegetables marinate for 30 minutes to an hour before grilling or broiling.

Spicy Orange & Cilantro

- 2 tablespoons olive oil
- 1 tablespoon orange juice
- 1 tablespoon orange marmalade
- 1 tablespoon chopped fresh cilantro
- 1 teaspoon red pepper flakes

Asian

- 2 tablespoons light soy sauce
- 2 tablespoons seasoned rice wine vinegar
- 2 teaspoons minced fresh ginger
- 1 teaspoon sesame oil

Brown Sugar & Bourbon

- 2 tablespoons soy sauce
- 2 tablespoons bourbon
- 1 tablespoon brown sugar
- 1 teaspoon cayenne pepper

Lemon & Garlic

- 1 tablespoon olive oil
- 2 tablespoons lemon juice
- 1 tablespoon lemon zest
- 1 teaspoon minced garlic
- Salt and freshly ground pepper to taste

Maple & Wasabi

- 2 tablespoons maple syrup
- 2 tablespoons olive oil
- 1 teaspoon wasabi

STEP

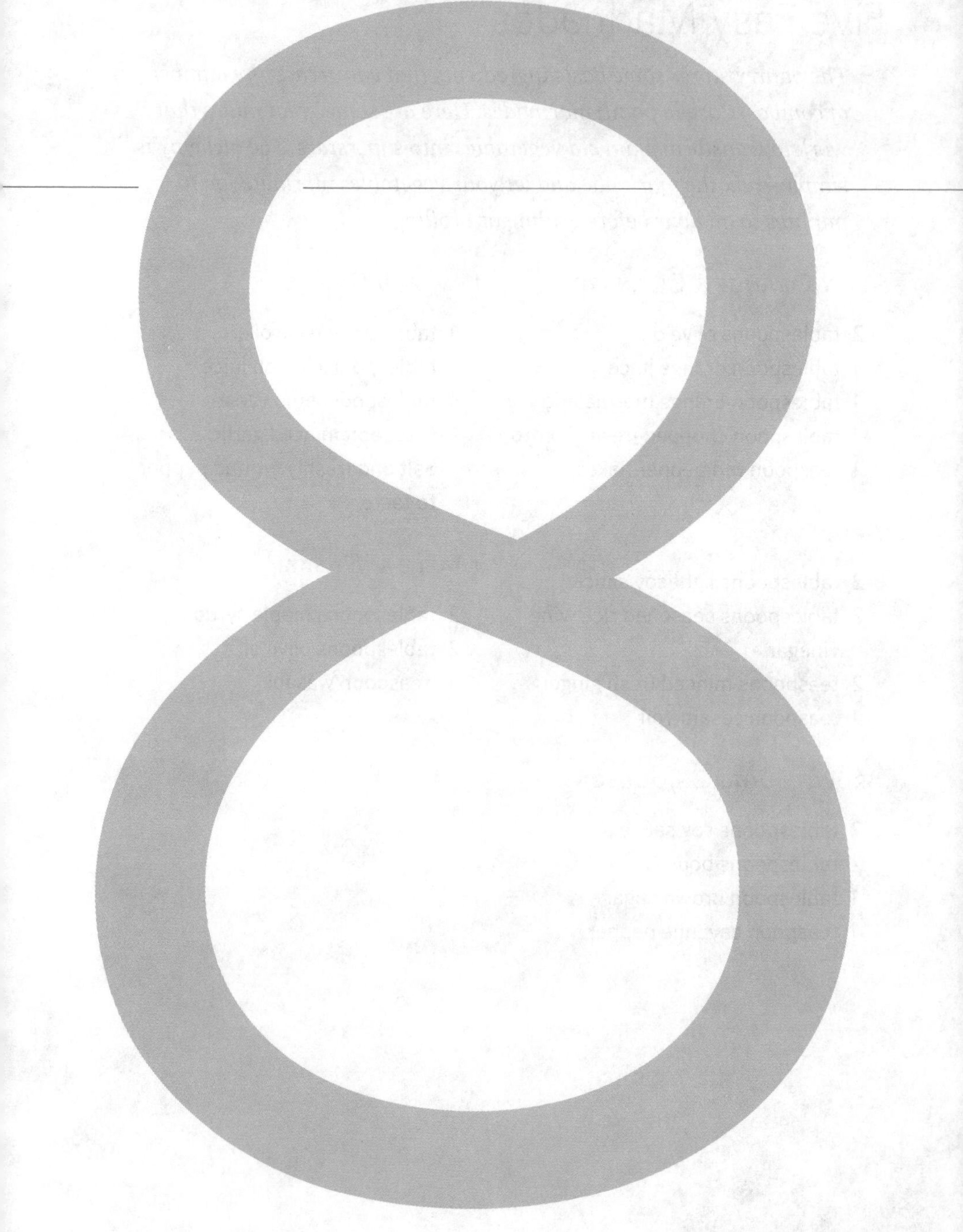

Green Your Kitchen

The hearth—even the modern equivalent with a metal stovetop—is always the center of our homes, a place that nourishes and nurtures and even promotes well-being. This chapter is all about finding ways to bring the highest purpose of the kitchen back into our lives. True food, prepared with love and care in an ecologically friendly and welcoming space, is the backdrop for richer lives and relationships.

WHAT IT MEANS

Health of the Household

Choose carefully what comes into and goes out of your kitchen.

Wendell Berry, in his book *Home Economics,* reminds us that in the original Greek, economics—*oikonomikos*—means "house" plus "steward" or "manager." Sharing the same root, *oikos,* the word "ecology" is closely related in concept—it is the relationships among organisms who share the same home. Thus, as Berry explains, a most important measure of the health of the planet is the health of its households.

Carefully choosing what enters and leaves the kitchen is, in every sense, to steward the health of the household and, in turn, the planet. All of us bring food, packaging, cleaning products, building materials, appliances, and more into our homes. Many of us also pour toxic cleaning products down drains, put packaging in landfills and incinerators, throw broken refrigerators into dumps—the list goes on. All of this has an impact on the environment and on our health. By monitoring the products brought into our homes, using them wisely, and disposing of them responsibly, we can, in the words of Wendell Berry, "make ourselves responsibly at home in the world."

TRUE TIP

Beeswax candles have the longest, cleanest burn of any candle; compared to paraffin candles made from polluted petroleum sludge, they are much more desirable. When beeswax candles burn, they emit negative ions, making them a natural air cleaner.

WHY IT MATTERS FOR YOU

A Healthful Kitchen

It's more than the food prepared there.

Kitchens are natural gathering spots for family and friends, a place to share good food, good talk, and good times. But they are more than just food; a healthful kitchen is as important as the goodness of the food brought into it.

We spend 90 percent of our time indoors, according to the EPA, and so our indoor air should be as clean as possible. Yet concentrations of many volatile organic compounds (VOCs) are up to ten times higher indoors than out. Study after scientific study demonstrates that exposing our children to even low levels of the toxic chemicals in common household products can contribute to health risks—from increasing asthma and allergies to promoting cancer to causing birth defects, developmental delays, and learning disorders. Reducing our exposure to toxic cleaning products, pesticides, and other commonly used household chemicals can have a dramatic impact on indoor air quality. Making responsible choices—to benefit the health of our families, friends, community, and ultimately the planet—is the process that leads to establishing a green kitchen.

WHY IT MATTERS FOR EARTH

The Hazards of Waste

Replace toxic household products with greener ones.

Just as more sustainable farms protect the local environment for all residents, so too do homes where you live efficiently, save energy and water, and reduce waste. A typical community the size of Bloomfield, Michigan—about 42,000 people—sends two tons of toilet bowl cleaner and seven tons of liquid household cleaner through the water system each month. Landfills, storm drains, and sewage treatment plants are not designed to treat chemical wastes. The chemicals may stay in the environment and move into drinking water supplies.

Your home doesn't have to be a part of this. Substitute easy-to-make nontoxic cleaning formulas for toxic ones. You'll be in good company: Most household hazardous waste websites offer alternatives. Green products on the market today work for any job in your home.

Consider as well the appliances in your kitchen. New energy-saving appliances can go a long way to reducing your carbon footprint. The average refrigerator manufactured in 2003 uses only 500 kilowatt-hours of electricity per year, while those manufactured in 1972 used more than 2,500.

And think of taking your produce scraps out to the compost heap instead of to the trash. Scraps in compost decompose into a rich, dark dirt that can be spread on your garden.

Simple Stewardship

HOUSEHOLD HAZARDOUS WASTE

Products such as paints, cleaners, oils, batteries, and pesticides, which contain potentially hazardous ingredients—and require special care when you dispose of them—don't belong in the kitchen. These products contain corrosive, toxic, ignitable, or reactive ingredients and are considered "household hazardous waste."

Hazardous waste includes:

- Cleaning products such as furniture polishes and stains, floor waxes, car waxes, spray dust cleaners, drain cleaners, toilet bowl cleaners, oven clean ers, petroleum-based spot and stain removers, all aerosols, and shoe polish
- Auto maintenance products such as motor oil, transmission fluid and additives, engine lubricants, antifreeze, windshield wiper solution, lead-acid batteries, engine cleaners and solvents, gas treatments, gas line freeze-up products, and car waxes
- Outside use products such as fertilizers, pesticides, pool chemicals, self-lighting charcoal, charcoal lighter fluid, butane lighters, hobby and repair products, paintbrush cleaner, sprays and aerosols, lacquers and thinners, alcohol (not for human consumption), creosote, naphtha, mineral spirits, turpentine, wood preservatives, glues and adhesives, and photographic chemicals

Improper disposal of household hazardous wastes can include pouring them down the drain, on the ground, into storm sewers, or in some cases putting them out with the trash. Hazardous waste in the garbage leaches into landfills and ultimately into the water supply; incinerated waste releases toxins into the air.

HOW TO DO IT

True Cleaning

Don't be overwhelmed by the challenge of greening your kitchen; take it one step at a time.

Greening a kitchen takes place on several fronts. Before you know it, an holistic approach happens naturally. Remove all of your household hazardous waste and refrain from buying anything as toxic ever again. Read labels about cleaning ingredients and gravitate toward simple and safe do-it-yourself formulas. Replace plastic and never buy it again.

Onward!

You can radically improve the indoor air quality of your home by simply switching to greener cleaning products. Use natural materials such as the minerals in baking soda, and acids in vinegar or lemon juice—materials with chemical properties that lend themselves to cleaning. Using updated versions of old cleaning formulas makes it easy to avoid toxic, synthetic cleaning agents.

A wide range of less toxic and biodegradable ready-made commercial cleaning products is increasingly

Vanilla is an age-old odor remover. Today we can use either the whole vanilla bean or natural vanilla extract. Place either 1-2 teaspoons of vanilla extract or 1 quartered vanilla bean in ¼ cup vodka poured into a teacup, and leave it in the open air. Make sure the vanilla extract isn't artificial or it won't do the trick.

If it can't be reduced, reused, repaired, rebuilt, refurbished, refinished, resold, recycled or composted, then it should be restricted, redesigned, or removed from production.

—PETE SEEGER, "IF IT CAN'T BE REDUCED"

available in health food stores and green supermarkets. The green cleaning product category is highly scrutinized, and the products found in health food stores tend to live up to their claims of being environmentally preferable. Some stores even offer brands in refillable containers. Natural cleaners can be substituted for cleaning products such as furniture polishes and stains, floor waxes, car waxes, spray dust cleaners, drain cleaners, toilet bowl cleaners, oven cleaners, petroleum-based spot and stain removers, all aerosols, and shoe polish.

Learning to clean from scratch by using cleansers made from kitchen cupboard ingredients can truly work if you take time to understand a bit about the chemistry behind how materials such as the minerals in baking soda and acids in lemon juice work. Another key to success is to choose the right materials for the right job.

TRUE TIP

Many communities in the United States offer a variety of options for conveniently and safely managing hazardous household waste. Learn more at the EPA's waste site: *www.epa.gov/epawaste/index.htm.*

BAKING SODA This miraculous mineral, sodium bicarbonate, has more uses for household cleaning than any other substance. It is made from soda ash, which is produced from a naturally occurring ore called trona, mined—by deep mining rather than more damaging strip mining—in Wyoming. Baking soda is slightly alkaline, with a pH around 8.1 (7 is neutral), so it neutralizes acid-based odors in water. Sprinkled on a damp sponge or cloth, baking soda can be used as a gentle cleaner for kitchen countertops. It is also a good scouring powder for sinks and bathtubs when combined with a dab of all-purpose detergent, and an excellent oven cleaner. It is gentle enough to be used to clean fiberglass.

Baking soda absorbs odors from the air—as many know who place an open box in the fridge. It is also a fine carpet deodorizer: Sprinkle it onto carpets and vacuum an hour later. Baking soda can even help keep drainpipes clear. When you pour baking soda and boiling water down a drain, you alter the soda's chemical composition, making it more caustic, and thus more effective in breaking down grease and dirt.

WASHING SODA A chemical cousin of baking soda, washing soda, or sodium carbonate, is more strongly alkaline, with a pH around 11. It is mined much like baking soda but processed differently. Because it is quite caustic, it cannot be called nontoxic; wear rubber gloves when using it. But it releases no harmful fumes and is far safer than a commercial solvent.

Fun, Kids, Pleasure

FRESHER SEASONAL AIR FRESHENERS

A study by the California Air Resources Board found that many household cleaners and plug-in air fresheners emit chemicals that, when combined with ozone, produce pollutants including formaldehyde, a known human carcinogen and a respiratory irritant. Instead of choosing such products, simmer a handful of seasonal herbs or spices.

FALL AND WINTER

The smell of apple cider mulled with cinnamon is an aroma of autumn that makes people feel warm and welcomed.

2 sticks or more of cinnamon
5 or 6 whole cloves
8 cups apple cider and water

Combine all the ingredients in a pan on the stove. Bring to a boil, then turn down to a simmer. Replace the liquid as needed, since it will evaporate.

SPRING AND SUMMER

Mint is a wonderful freshener that has antiviral and antibacterial properties. Some say it enhances concentration. Use either fresh or dried mint in this formula.

A handful of mint leaves (or 4-5 mint tea bags)
8 cups of water

Combine all the ingredients in a pan on the stove. Bring to a boil, and then turn down to a simmer. Replace the liquid when needed as it evaporates.

Washing soda is a real find for natural cleaning because it is a powerful, heavy-duty cleaner. It cuts grease, cleans petroleum oils and dirt, removes wax or lipstick, and softens water. It will clean a petroleum spill on the basement or garage floor. It can be made into scouring powders and soft scrubbers, floor cleaners, and all-purpose cleaners. Traditionally used as a laundry detergent booster, it works well for that job, too. It also neutralizes odors as baking soda does. Washing soda is too caustic to use on fiberglass, aluminum, or waxed floors—unless you intend to remove the wax. For heavy-duty jobs, make washing soda into a thick paste with water; apply, scrub, and rinse well. For less intensive jobs, mix one-half to one cup of washing soda per gallon of water. (Warm water is needed to dissolve the washing soda.)

Healthy for You

WORDS OF WARNING

There are few government safeguards in place regarding the safety of commercial cleaning products, but "signal words" on product labels are one notable exception. They are placed there by order of the federal government to help protect you and your family. Learn how to recognize the warnings alerting you to toxic products.

- **POISON/DANGER** means something very toxic; only a few drops could kill you.
- **WARNING** means moderately toxic; as little as a teaspoonful can kill.
- **CAUTION** denotes a product that is less toxic; two tablespoons to a cup could kill you.
- **OTHER WARNING WORDS** include Strong, Sensitizer, Toxic, Carcinogen, Flammable, and Corrosive.

Simple Stewardship

WHAT'S UNDER YOUR KITCHEN SINK?

Almost everyone in the U.S. has a cupboard full of poisons under the kitchen sink. Wasp spray, oven cleaner, waxes and polishes—the place is full of chemicals that display words such as poison, danger, warning, or caution. Removing these products from under the kitchen sink is recommended. Small amounts of the poisons drift from and leak out of containers and spray bottles and can waft around the kitchen. Household poisonings are one of the greatest threats to children. Place products with signal words in a locked cupboard in an out-of-the-way place such as a garage. Once you have removed the toxic chemicals, you can make a fresh start with nonpolluting, biodegradable alternative products.

WHITE DISTILLED VINEGAR White distilled vinegar and lemon juice are the opposites of baking and washing soda: They are acidic and so neutralize alkaline, or caustic, substances. Vinegar kills germs, bacteria, and viruses. Numerous studies show that a straight 5 percent solution of vinegar—the kind you can buy in the supermarket—kills 99 percent of bacteria, 82 percent of mold, and 80 percent of germs (viruses). Kitchen maven Heloise also reports similar results from tests. If your tap water is hard and you have trouble with mineral buildup (scale), soak a cloth in vinegar and rest it on the scale buildup for a few hours. The acid will break down the minerals and they can be wiped away. Acids dissolve gummy buildup and eat away tarnish. Vinegar is also particularly good for removing dirt from wood surfaces.

LIQUID SOAPS AND DETERGENTS Liquid soaps and detergents are necessary for washing dishes, windows, and floors. Detergents are synthetic materials made up of surfactants (surface active agents), which are derived from vegetable oils, animal fats, or petroleum constituents. Discovered and synthesized early in this century, detergents are considered an improvement over soap because they don't react with hard-water minerals. This protects clothes from getting gray and prevents soap scum and film from forming on tiles, tubs, and sinks.

The brands of liquid soaps and detergents that are the purest—without dyes, perfumes, and other additives—are primarily found in health food stores. If you have hard water, buy a detergent; if you have soft water, you can use a real soap.

DISINFECTANTS For a substance to be registered by the EPA as a disinfectant, it must go through extensive and expensive tests; the product is then registered as a pesticide. Many of the disinfectants registered contain chemicals that can cause the same problem as overuse of antibiotics, or superbug overgrowth. Superbugs are a hazard in kitchens, especially with the sick or elderly who have compromised immune systems.

Healthy for You

SPONGES

Almost every sponge now sold in U.S. supermarkets is impregnated with a synthetic disinfectant—usually triclosan— registered as a pesticide with the EPA. Avoid washing your dishes and countertops with chemicals that leave a residue.

Instead, buy pure cellulose sponges and avoid sponges in packages that use language such as "kills odors." Sterilize sponges by boiling them in a pan of water for three to five minutes, or wash them in a dishwasher with a load of dishes.

Australian Tea Tree Oil

Australian tea tree oil and grapefruit seed extract are two ingredients that folk legend claims kill bacteria and mold, in addition to acting as successful disinfectants. While not registered with the EPA as disinfectants, they do work well for killing mold and mildew. Australian tea tree oil is an essential oil from the melaleuca tree. It has a strong but not unpleasant odor that dissipates after a few days. Though this oil is expensive, a little bit goes a long way. A grapefruit seed-extract spray can be made by adding 20 drops of extract to a quart of water. Both Australian tea tree oil and grapefruit seed extract are available in health food stores.

To clean the sink, simply pour about half a cup of baking soda into a corner of the sink, and slowly add liquid detergent, stirring while you add, until the mixture has a texture like frosting. Scoop the mixture onto a sponge, and wash the sink. Rinse.

Chemical-Free Disinfectants

- Botanical Disinfectants

  Look for botanical disinfectants as there are a few registered by the EPA as hospital-grade disinfectants, achieving a 100 percent kill rate, yet they don't cause superbug overgrowth. Benefect Botanical Disinfectant is one brand.

- Dry Vapor Steam

  Steam cleaners disinfect by using only water to dry steam at levels of 240°F and above. While expensive, they are chemical free.

- UV SterilizingTool

  For an all-purpose sterilizing method that uses no chemicals yet has a 99.9 percent kill rate, consider UV sterilizing equipment, such as the Purelight UV Sterilizing Wand sold by Gaiam. It kills not only viruses, bacteria, and mold but also dust mites and bed bugs.

Do-It-Yourself Cleaning Formulas

You'll find DIY cleaning formulas in this chapter—effective cleaning agents made with safe, basic ingredients.

We suggest you mix and match with a few commercial green products, such as a good all-purpose detergent and a few essential oils to your liking.

ALKALINE CLEANER This formula is the basic all-purpose cleaner to have on hand for cleaning baseboards, walls, counters, and similar jobs.

½ teaspoon washing soda
½ teaspoon liquid soap or detergent
2 cups hot water or club soda (rich in alkaline minerals)

Combine all the ingredients in a spray bottle, making sure that the water is hot enough to dissolve the minerals. Shake to blend. Use as you would a normal all-purpose spray cleanser.
MAKES 2 cups
COST $0.07 (cost of leading commercial cleaner: $1.51)
NOTE: Takes about 1 minute to prepare; shelf life is indefinite.

ACID CLEANER Acid cleaners are very helpful for scale (mineral buildup), and pet and body odors.

¼ cup white distilled vinegar or lemon juice
½ teaspoon liquid wool detergent
¾ cup warm water

Combine the ingredients in a spray bottle. Shake to blend before use.
MAKES 1 cup
COST $0.06 (cost of leading commercial cleaner: $0.75)
NOTE: Takes about 1 minute to prepare; shelf life is indefinite with vinegar, a few days for lemon juice. Store in the refrigerator.

OVEN CLEANER Most people don't know that simple household minerals such as baking soda clean like magic. The key is using enough. To clean your oven, sprinkle baking soda all over the bottom until it is covered completely with about one-fourth inch baking soda. Then, using a clean spray bottle, spray the baking soda with water until the baking soda is thoroughly damp but not flooded. After that, go off and do other things. When you think of it, dampen the baking soda again if it is drying out. Before you go to bed, do that again. When you wake up in the morning, the baking soda can effortlessly be scooped out of the oven with a sponge, bringing all the grime with it, and leaving no fumes behind. That's it! The only downside is that you need to rinse out the white residue left by the baking soda.

Simple Stewardship

SOFT SCRUBBER FOR STAINLESS STEEL

The bane of stainless steel owners seems to be streaks and fingerprints. New stainless steel is protected for a number of years by a chromium film that protects the metal from rusting, staining, and even tarnishing. But if you don't keep up with the stains, the film can be compromised and repair becomes difficult.

For everyday cleanup as well as the more heavy-duty jobs, try this. Place ½ cup baking soda in a bowl and add enough green liquid soap or detergent to make a texture like frosting. Scoop some of the mixture onto a sponge and scrub the stainless steel. Rinse well.

After cleaning with this, some people like to bring the stainless steel to a high polish by rubbing the surface with straight household vinegar. But just rinsing the soft-scrub well does the trick.

NOTE: Stay away from all chlorine-based products on stainless steel.

Simple Stewardship

ALL-PURPOSE CLEANER FOR BIG JOBS

EVERYDAY FORMULA

If you are inspired to wash walls, or have some big cleaning project, this preparation will be useful. It makes 2 gallons, takes about 4 minutes to prepare, and costs 62 cents; the leading commercial cleaner costs $31.92.

¼ cup each washing soda and liquid soap or detergent
2 gallons hot water

Combine the ingredients in a pail and stir to dissolve. Wearing gloves, saturate a sponge with the mixture, wring out the excess liquid, and wash the area. Resaturate the sponge frequently as you go. Rinse well.

HEAVY-DUTY FORMULA

Use this for tough stains and grease, such as engine oil. This formula makes 1 cup. It takes about a minute to prepare. It costs about 6 cents; the leading commercial grease remover costs $6.50.

2 teaspoons washing soda
½ teaspoon liquid soap or detergent
1 cup hot water

Combine the ingredients in a spray bottle and shake well. Spray the stain. The high concentration of washing soda can result in white residue, so rinse well with water. Wipe dry.

APPLIANCE CLEANER This basic formula can clean all the appliances in your kitchen.

½ teaspoon washing soda
2 teaspoons liquid soap
2 cups hot tap water

Combine in a clean spray bottle. Shake well to dissolve. **NOTE:** Variations on this formula can include substituting vinegar (this can double as a window cleaner) or borax for the washing soda.

Water

The human body is mostly water—our cells are 75 to 90 percent water—so it stands to reason that clean water is a critical component of good health.

SAVING WATER Humans are a thirsty lot; in the U.S. each person uses an average of 70 gallons per day—and that's just indoors. It can be hard to think about saving water, since it's always there when you turn on the tap. But we could all cut down on our water consumption, especially during hot, dry summers. Droughts across the country are depleting municipal water supplies, and in 2007, at the height of the dry season in August, as much as 42 percent of the country across 29 of the 50 states experienced a drought.

As municipal water supplies dry up, costs increase. So saving water is like saving money; fortunately, there are ways to save water and keep it clean and healthful without forking over money for new water-saving appliances.

Faucet Fixes

Worried about what's in your water because of old pipes, so you run the tap to flush out the heavy metals and sediments? Instead, install a water filtration system in the basement or under the sink; it will remove problem metals and chemicals in your water. Here are more ideas on how to troubleshoot your home's water issues.

- Got a leaky faucet? Fix it. A dripping faucet can waste 75 gallons of water a week. Call a plumber if you can't fix it yourself.
- Install an aerator on your faucet. This inexpensive attachment mixes air into the water as it leaves the tap. While not affecting the volume or pressure, an aerator can reduce a water flow of four to five gallons a minute to two and a half gallons a minute.

- A garbage disposal uses up about two to seven gallons of water per minute, so only run it when full. Composting is a more ecological choice for food waste.

BOTTLED WATER Ditch bottled water. It takes three liters of water to produce one liter of bottled water, thanks to all the resources needed to make a plastic bottle. Further, the privatization of the water supply has made it legal for corporations to cross borders and plunder the water they find. And the plastics from the bottles can leach into the water. This is especially problematic for water bottled in polycarbonate plastic.

Bottled water companies, whose products come under the jurisdiction of the Food and Drug Administration (FDA), are not required to report water contaminants. By contrast, municipalities are required to report dangerous chemicals or bacteria within 24 hours. The FDA doesn't even know which food manufacturers produce bottled water, a vivid assessment of how unregulated bottled water is. During the summer of 2009,

Healthy for You

WASH HANDS WITH SOAP AND WATER

Washing hands is an essential way to reduce germs. Avoid hand cleansers with antimicrobial chemicals due to potential health risks. The EPA recommends killing germs by washing with soapy water. Make sure you buy a real soap, as some products that call themselves a soap are actually detergents, and unlikely to work as well as a real, alkaline soap. (Many detergents are closer to a neutral pH.) Dr. Bronner's liquid castile soap is a real soap, or find handmade bar soaps in health food stores. Those with essential oils will also offer some extra antimocrobial protection.

the Government Accountability Office urged the FDA to require bottlers to use labels that would, at the least, tell consumers how to get comprehensive information. Consumption of bottled water totaled 28.5 gallons per person in the U.S. in 2008, nearly double the amount in 1998.

WASHING DISHES In terms of water use, a full dishwasher uses less water than hand washing. *Consumer Reports* advises against rinsing before loading. Pre-rinsing doesn't help clean your dishes and it's a big waste of water—up to 20 gallons per load. Scrape food into the garbage, or better yet, compost it.

Choose a powder dishwasher detergent: Water-based detergents are heavier than dried detergents, and the extra weight of the product means more energy and cost to transport.

If you have tried green automatic dishwasher detergent in the past, try it again. The research and development teams of green companies such as Seventh Generation, Eco-One, and Ecover have worked hard to make phosphate-free products work, and they are succeeding.

If you hand-wash your dishes, you can save five gallons of water (or as much as a third of what you otherwise would need), according to David Goldbeck in *Smart Kitchen,* by "ponding" water. To pond for hand washing dishes, fill the sink with water, and wash the dishes in the full sink, instead of washing the dishes under a stream of water. If you have side-by-side sinks, fill both sides with water; wash in one and rinse in the other. For washing dishes by hand, choose a green liquid dish detergent that is free of perfumes and dyes.

SAFE WATER More than 260 contaminants are found in U.S. drinking water, according to a 2005 study of tap water in 42 states by the Environmental Working Group (EWG). No enforceable safety limits were found in 140 of the contaminants, while 116 of those found had safety standards. The group found tap water contaminated with 83 agricultural pollutants, including pesticides and fertilizer ingredients, in the water of 201,955,000 people in 41 states. Water contaminated with 166 industrial pollutants, including plasticizers, solvents, and propellants, are in the water of 210,528,000 people in 42 states.

Bacteria and viruses from sewage can commonly seep into wells. If you are on a municipal water system, law requires that water be disinfected with chlorine. The Safe Drinking Water Act of 1974—primarily overseen by the EPA and amended a number of times, lastly in 1996—requires your municipality to test for possible contaminants. As of 2003, 95 water contaminants were regulated by the U.S. Environmental Protection Agency. Some contaminants are not tested, and many people wish to remove the taste of chlorine from their water. Filtering household water is increasingly desirable, no matter where you may live.

Buying spring water in plastic gallon jugs is not the answer for an ecological kitchen, however. Buying a $300 whole-house water filter is cheaper by half than the yearly cost of the equivalent amount of water in plastic jugs. Further, plastic jugs cost the environment dearly, even if they are recyclable in your community. Water in plastic gallon jugs is not regulated in a way that insures safe water, and the plastic can leach into the water. Larger water jugs made of polycarbonate contain endocrine disrupters.

CARBON FILTERS Activated carbon filters are the most common filters on the market. They work to purify water because they absorb contaminants, and as the water passes through the carbon, suspended solids are filtered and trapped by the carbon. Carbon filters can reduce chlorine and some man-made chemicals, including chlordane, benzene, and carbon tetrachloride; some filters reduce lead. Carbon filters are available in sizes and styles that range from whole-house treatment to small pour-through pitchers. Carbon filter cartridges need to be replaced regularly.

ALERT Carbon filters will not remove bacteria or viruses. Some experts recommend carbon filters only be used on municipal water supplies that are continually disinfected with chlorine. Silver-impregnated carbon filters slow the growth of bacteria but do not kill bacteria already in the water.

REVERSE OSMOSIS In reverse osmosis, water is filtered first through a cartridge that removes suspended solids, and then through a membrane that can reduce heavy metals such as lead, mercury, and arsenic; bacteria and viruses; and pesticides and herbicides.

ALERT In reverse osmosis, the water comes in contact with a lot of plastic, and some people complain that at first the water tastes of plastic. Also, for each gallon of purified drinking water, you will waste four gallons of water. While this is wasteful enough, systems that do not have shut-off

Healthy for You

CLEANING CUTTING BOARDS

Do not use cutting boards for animal products. (Cut them on plates and wash the plates in an automatic dishwasher.) Whenever you use a cutting board, scrub it well with soap and water, rinse, and then spray it with straight white distilled vinegar and don't rinse. Alternatively, spray with a lavender spray, and don't rinse. (To make a lavender spray, combine 1 teaspoon of a pure essential oil of lavender in a clean spray bottle with 1 cup of water; shake to blend.)

valves continue to waste water when the storage tank is full. Most contemporary reverse osmosis systems have a shut-off valve—make sure before buying one.

What is your water's pH? The higher the pH, the more minerals it has. Minerals are good for the heart, but water with too many minerals can taste off. Mineral-laden water can also require more detergent and whiteners to clean clothes and dishes, and it can create soap scum. Ideally, water should have a pH between 6 and 8.5.

DISTILLATION Distillers produce the purest water—so pure that all its health-promoting minerals have been removed. Still, distillation reduces chemicals, heavy metals, and bacteria and viruses by 90 percent or more. Distillers work by boiling water, turning it into steam, and cooling it again to a liquid state. Contaminants are left behind in the steam or boiling tank. Most distillers also contain a carbon filter to reduce any volatile organic chemicals present that may not be reduced in the distiller's boiling or steam stage because their boiling point is similar to water. **ALERT** Distillers require a lot of electricity to operate. Water-cooled distillers use more water than air-cooled distillers. Choose distillers made of stainless steel, not aluminum, since small amounts of aluminum may leach into the water with unknown health effects. Last but not least, distillers reduce vital minerals such as

Healthy for You

HERE'S TO HEALTHY FAUCETS

Faucets can be sources of lead, cadmium, mercury, and other toxic substances. The EPA, the plumbing industry, and public health officials have recently developed standards for how much lead and other toxics a faucet can contribute to the water. Six manufacturers have passed the tests. (Passing means that lead can contribute no more than 11 parts per billion to the lead content of the water.) Look for the NSF International logo on boxes of faucets when you buy them. NSF International is the company that carried out the tests, and you can check out their website at *www.nsf.org* for a full list of approved faucets.

magnesium from the water supply, and while water is not the only source of these minerals, a healthful diet must make up for their loss in drinking water.

Energy Use in the Kitchen

There is a lot at stake in our use of kitchen appliances. According to David Goldbeck in *Smart Kitchen,* some 20 to 40 percent of household energy is consumed in the kitchen. If you are in the market for a new kitchen appliance, pay attention to EnergyGuide labels, required by federal law on most new kitchen appliances. Each label will offer information about the manufacturer and details such as model number, comparative energy efficiency, estimated energy consumption in kilowatt-hours per year (kWh/year), and estimated annual energy costs.

SMALL KITCHEN A green kitchen cluttered with small appliances seems a contradiction in terms, yet small appliances use less energy for specialized cooking jobs than big electric appliances.

Baking four potatoes in a toaster oven makes more sense from an energy standpoint than baking the potatoes in a full-size oven, for example. An electric teapot takes less energy than heating a teakettle on the stove, as does using a rice cooker, a crock pot, or an electric fry pan. The reason for this is that the heating element is built right into the small appliance and transfers the heat more efficiently. Microwaves are extremely energy-efficient because the source of energy is from electromagnetic waves, not heat. Instead of being consumer indulgences, small appliances are energy savers.

REFRIGERATORS AND FREEZERS These appliances are the biggest energy users in the kitchen. Up-to-date refrigerators are significantly more energy-efficient than their older counterparts, saving up to 50 percent in energy costs. Here are some guidelines for choosing and maintaining energy-efficient refrigerators and freezers.

- Side-by-side refrigerator/freezers use up to 13 percent more energy than a typical refrigerator with the freezer above or below it.
- Automatic ice makers increase energy use.
- The ideal temperature for a refrigerator is 38°F to 40°F; 0°F to 5°F for a freezer. Place a thermometer inside the refrigerator to monitor the temperature.
- Make sure that the door gaskets are not ripped or broken in any way.
- Try to place a freezer in as cool a room as possible. A chest freezer is more energy-efficient than an upright, because less warm air enters when it opens.
- Keep the top of the refrigerator uncluttered.
- The fuller a freezer, the more energy-efficient.
- Don't place hot foods in the refrigerator or freezer. Cool them to room temperature first.
- Open fridge or freezer doors as little as possible.
- Make sure the refrigerator or freezer is not in the direct sun, or next to the stove.

DISHWASHERS Eighty percent of the cost of running a dishwasher is in heating the water, reports David Goldbeck in *Smart Kitchen.* But as with refrigerators, there are ways to reduce the amount of energy consumption.

- The hot water used for dishwashers must reach 140°F to remove grease and dissolve detergent. In older dishwasher models the hot water heater for the whole house has to be set at that high temperature, which is very costly in energy use. Most new dishwashers, however, have a special booster heater to heat the water for the dishwasher alone to the specified 140°F, making it possible to keep the temperature of the house's hot water heater at 120°F instead.

- Use the air-dry option. Better yet, open the door of the dishwasher for that last drying cycle.
- Use the shortest dishwashing cycle. Only run a full load.
- Rinse the dishes as little as possible before loading.

STOVES There are many options for stoves. Here are guidelines on how choices affect home energy use.

- Induction cooktops—the kind with a ceramic surface, like a countertop—are the most energy-efficient.
- Convection ovens are the most energy-efficient because heated air is continuously circulated.

Shopping & Saving

LUNCH BOX ENLIGHTENMENT

Stainless steel lunch boxes, lead-free cloth lunch bags, reusable lunch napkins, stainless steel water bottles, vinyl/PVC-free insulated lunch bags. Renovations in lunch box ware all add up to save you a lot of money and the world a lot of resources. Check out:

- Laptop Lunch Boxes (*www.laptoplunches.com*)
- To-Go Ware (*www.to-goware.com*)
- Reusable Bags (*www.reusablebags.com*)

Also, take inspiration from the Edible Schoolyard, a one-acre garden and kitchen classroom at Martin Luther King, Jr., Middle School in Berkeley, California. The garden started as a cover crop in a vacant lot, tended once monthly by students. More than a decade later, it is a thriving acre of vegetables, fruits, herbs, and flowers.

The Edible Schoolyard is a program of the Chez Panisse Foundation, a nonprofit organization founded by chef and author Alice Waters. Learn about the program and other resources on the website: *www.edibleschoolyard.org.*

Gas stoves are more energy-efficient than electric, but they do cause indoor air pollution. New gas stoves with electronic ignition use around 30 percent less gas than those with a pilot light. Upgrade to an electronic ignition model if you can. To make sure a gas stove is working efficiently, check the flame: It should be bluish. If it is yellow, call the gas company to have the stove adjusted.

Cooking Tips to Save Energy

- Match the pan to the size of the heating coil.
- Cover pans when cooking.
- Turn off the burner or oven before the food is completely cooked.
- Low-fat and low-liquid cooking reduces cooking time.
- Reheat leftovers on top of the range, not in the oven.
- Use a pressure cooker whenever possible.
- Invest in an electric slow cooker, the most energy-efficient system of cooking, next to a microwave.
- Make more food than you need; freeze the rest for your own "fast food."
- Try cooking in one pot to minimize energy expenditure—for yourself as well as the stove.
- If you eat a lot of pasta, cook a week's worth at once, toss lightly in oil, and keep in the refrigerator.

LIGHTING Lighting accounts for about 15 percent of household energy use. Incandescent bulbs are inefficient, because a lot of energy is wasted as heat. Compact fluorescent bulbs are 75 percent more efficient. If every household in America switched to compact fluorescent bulbs in only one room, power plants would release one trillion pounds less CO_2—the major greenhouse gas—into the atmosphere each year.

Shopping & Saving

KITCHEN ECONOMICS

Take the example of substituting cloth towels for paper towels. At an upstate New York supermarket, recycled paper towels cost $2.00 for 175 sheets. An average family goes through 96 rolls a year at a cost of $192. In comparison, 12 cotton towels would last about three years, at a cost of $35. For that period you would have spent $576 on paper towels; buying cotton towels would save $541.

Compact fluorescents for every kind of fixture are available in most hardware stores. Be sure you use EnergyStar compact fluorescents, tested for quality and longevity.

Washing dishes in an automatic dishwasher is the most effective way to sanitize them. A recent study revealed a hand-washed plate with a count of 390 bacteria, compared with a plate washed in a dishwasher with hot water heated to at least 130°F, with a bacteria count of 1.

PHANTOM LOADS "Phantom" energy, the power drawn by equipment left on and digital dials left blinking, can account for 8 percent of a household's annual electricity use and cost some $80 per year. Add in seldom-used appliances that drain energy through their plugs, and the monthly total could double. *Home Power* magazine estimates that the electricity represented by such phantom loads in the United States equals the total electricity used in Greece, Peru, and Vietnam combined. Our advice:

- Unplug seldom-used appliances, like the refrigerator in the basement or garage that contains just a few items.
- Unplug chargers that are not charging, and keep them unplugged until you need them.
- Use power strips to switch off televisions, home theater equipment, and stereos when you're not using them. Even when you think these products are off, together their standby consumption can be equivalent to a 75- or 100-watt light bulb running continuously.

Equipping the Green Kitchen

It's worth keeping track of your garbage for a few weeks. Watch what you throw away, and ask yourself if each item you are tossing could be replaced with a reusable substitute. You may see many coffee filters in the trash, for example. Why not buy a gold or cloth reusable coffee filter instead? You may see a lot of Popsicle wrappers. How about investing in good plastic molds to make your own? Or reusable sandwich boxes to replace plastic bags for lunches? Not only will you significantly reduce your consumption of resources by choosing reusable housewares instead of disposables, but you will also save a great deal of money.

TRUE TIP

The Environmental Defense Fund has details about the lead content of 8,000 china patterns. Visit their website to read their owner's guide and buyer's guides: ***www.edf.org/article.cfm?contentid=952***

IDEAS FOR REUSE

With reusable substitutes, you can cut back on plastic bags, wrap, and water jugs; aluminum foil; paper plates, cups, towels, and napkins; paper coffee filters, and more. We are all still faced with packaging waste to throw away, as well as worn-out items, but it may be surprising to learn how many items can be reused. Here are a few:

- Gold or cloth coffee filters, or use a French press pot
- Cloth towels
- Cloth napkins
- Durable metal plates and cups for picnics and birthday parties; reusable stainless steel utensils for picnics
- Reusable baking pans
- Cloth bags for shopping, including string bags for produce
- Reusable lunch box containers
- Glass mason jars with wide mouths and screw-on lids for food storage

HELPFUL EQUIPMENT There are many choices of kitchen appliances, gadgets, and gizmos available. Use those that make your cooking experience more convenient and energy efficient. You may or may not want a Crock-pot or bread-maker, for example, and whether you can buy special steel knives may be a matter of finances. But there are three important appliances that can make a big difference in producing flavorful, fresh, whole foods in your kitchen: a steamer for grains and vegetables, a pressure cooker, and a grinder for grains, spices, and nuts.

DINNERWARE WITHOUT LEAD Plates and dishes now sold in the United States are subject to federal regulations for the maximum amount of lead they may contain. The federal standards require that plates contain no more than 3 parts per million (ppm) of lead, and pitchers and other hollowware that hold liquid can contain no more than 0.5 ppm. California regulations require that no more than 0.2265 ppm of lead be found in dinnerware, and no more than 0.1 ppm in pitchers or hollowware.

Because major dinnerware manufacturers sell their dishes in California as well as the rest of the country, if you buy a major brand of dishes you can be assured

Simple Stewardship

REDUCE, RECYCLE, ESPECIALLY REUSE

Reusables surround you: Reuse glass condiment jars as containers in which to make salad dressings and marinades; reuse yogurt tubs for storing dry kitchen staples or for organizing hardware; reuse old cotton clothing and sheets for dusting and cleaning rags. (There's nothing like old, soft cotton for cleaning.)

Simple Stewardship

PAPER OR CLOTH?

Whether you rely on paper or cloth towels and napkins, there are a number of ways to make your choice a better option for the environment.

IF YOU USE PAPER TOWELS OR NAPKINS:

- Purchase paper towels made of 100 percent recycled materials and wound on 100 percent recycled core.
- Look for paper products that contain a minimum of 90 percent post-consumer waste.
- Choose unbleached paper towels. If those are unavailable, opt for process chlorine-free (PCF) next, or elemental chlorine-free (ECF) last.
- Choose paper towels and napkins that have no added pigments, inks, or dyes.
- Select packaging with minimal environmental impact, such as that made of recycled and recyclable materials and containing no toxic metals, dyes, or inks.
- Seek items having the largest amount of product to minimize packaging; for example, high-capacity hard-wound roll towels have 800 feet or more. Some brands are puffier and allow for fewer paper towels per roll or napkins per package.
- Avoid folded paper towels—it's too easy to use too many of them.

IF YOU USE CLOTH NAPKINS OR DISHTOWELS:

- Only wash when soiled. Most adults don't really dirty a napkin after every meal.
- Designate a place to store "in-use" napkins and use the same one until it is dirty.
- If you have a large family, designate a napkin ring for each member to identify their napkin between meals.
- Toss dirty napkins and dish towels in with other laundry. Use eco-friendly detergent.
- Wash with cold water and line dry whenever possible.

We owe much to the fruitful meditations of our sages, but a sane view of life is, after all, elaborated mainly in the kitchen.

— **JOSEPH CONRAD (1923)**

that they meet the stricter California regulations for lead content. Dinnerware is placed in a 4 percent acetic acid solution for 24 hours, and then the acid bath is tested for lead. Acidic substances extract lead, so be particularly cautious about storing juices and wines in containers that could have lead in them. The most serious concern is drinking liquid that has been stored in older lead crystal or older pewter. In pottery, the lead is in the glazes. When in doubt, ask if the glazed dinnerware you are considering is lead-free. Be particularly wary of bright red glazes.

POTS AND PANS When heated to between 680° and 930°F—scorching heat—the fluoropolymers used in chemical nonstick finishes degrade into several undesirable substances, including trifluoroacetate (TFA), a substance highly toxic to plants. Other problematic chemicals recently found in almost all blood samples taken by the Red Cross include perfluorinated acids and perfluorooctanic acid (PFOA), used in many nonstick and stainproof formulas. PFOA was found in the umbilical cord blood of 99 percent of 300 babies born at Johns Hopkins Hospital in 2004.

An independent scientific review panel advising the EPA recently announced that PFOA should be considered a likely carcinogen. In a voluntary agreement with the EPA, eight major manufacturers have agreed to eliminate 95 percent of PFOA emissions by 2010, though they will continue to use the chemical in making nonstick finishes. The nonprofit Environmental Working Group notes that at 680°F, nonstick finishes give off six toxic gases.

What to do? Get rid of all your coated nonstick pots and pans. But don't stop there. Be on the lookout for the nonstick chemical polytetrafluoroethylene (PTFE), used on cookware. Watch out for "nonstick" labeling and ask if the coating is PTFE, no matter what the brand. Most manufacturers offer a variety of different types of pots

Heavy cast-iron pans are nonstick when properly seasoned (lightly oiled and baked). Cast-iron pans hold heat, are inexpensive, add a little iron to your diet—and they're a joy to cook with. Just remember to replenish the seasoning of your cast-iron cookware by applying a thin layer of oil after each cleaning. Seasoning is an ongoing process, and the more you use cast iron, the more nonstick it becomes.

and pans. When you do replace your pans, choose cast iron, stainless steel, or enameled iron.

The Safest Pots and Pans

The more inert the cookware, the better. Use these:

- Glass—the most inert
- Stainless steel
- Well-seasoned cast iron
- Porcelain-coated cookware, also called enamel
- Anodized aluminum

Avoid these:

- Nonstick coated surfaces
- Aluminum (acidic foods can cause aluminum to leach from the pan)
- Plastic-handled cookware

KITCHEN CABINETS Kitchen cabinets are often made of particleboard coated with a wood veneer. The resin that glues the wood chips and sawdust in the particleboard together contains formaldehyde, considered a probable human carcinogen by the EPA. The veneer reduces formaldehyde emissions, but is often used only on the surface that faces the kitchen; the interior cabinet surfaces may be unfaced and capable of releasing the volatile form of formaldehyde. If you are buying new cabinets, consider those made of hard wood or metal instead of particleboard.

Concerned that your gas stove might be a safety hazard? Contact the Gas Appliance Manufacturers Association through their website: *www.agamanet. org.*

GAS STOVES While gas stoves are energy savers, they can cause a significant amount of indoor air pollution, in particular high indoor concentrations of nitrogen dioxide (NO_2) and carbon monoxide (CO). According to the EPA, NO_2 can cause increased risk of respiratory tract infection, chronic bronchitis, and increases in asthma. The EPA also notes that average levels of CO in homes without

Healthy for You

GRAIN GRINDER

Once grains—and many other foods such as spices and nuts—are milled, they lose a great deal of their nutritional value. And the longer between the milling of the grain, grinding of the spices, or chopping of the nuts, the more rancid the natural oils in the foods can get. Grinding your own flours will cost only a fraction of flours already ground. Further, the superb flavor of freshly ground grains, nuts, and spices bears no resemblance to anything that has been sitting on the shelf for a while.

gas stoves vary from 0.5 to 5 ppm. Levels near properly adjusted gas stoves are often 5 to 15 ppm, and those near poorly adjusted stoves may be 30 ppm or higher.

If you use a gas stove, make sure your stove has an automatic pilot and is well ventilated. It should have an exhaust hood and a fan to the outside, or at least you should keep a window open when using the stove. Upgrade to an appliance with electronic ignition instead of a pilot light. Never use your gas stove for heat. Never cook with charcoal inside the home.

If you have particleboard or pressed-wood cabinets, seal in the formaldehyde with AFM SafeCoat. For more on this product, visit the website: ***www.afmsafecoat.com.***

EXHAUST FANS A basic kitchen exhaust fan simply removes the smoke, filters it, and recirculates it in the kitchen, and a dirty fan and filter can become a fire hazard of built-up grease. Make sure your exhaust fan vents to the outside.

Pest Control

"A midnight encounter with a cockroach in your kitchen is enough to make even the staunchest environmentalist wish for a can of bug killer," writes science writer Catherine Zandonella. "To protect your family's and your planet's health, reach for a shoe instead. Pesticides are designed to kill bugs but they can have subtle but long-term effects on humans, especially the very young."

There are a number of less toxic ways of combating kitchen pests such as ants, flies, and roaches. The best resource of less toxic alternatives is the book *Common Sense Pest Control: Least Toxic Solutions for Your Home, Garden, Pets and Community.* It is an expensive book, but you can suggest your local library get it as a community service. The Rachel Carson Council *(www.rachelcarsoncouncil.org)* also offers publications that are pest-specific, with safe, practical ways to eradicate the pest in question.

ANTS In a bowl, mix 1 cup borax, 1 cup sugar, and 3 cups water. Place a loose wad of toilet paper into four different screw-top jars that are about the size of shallow marinated artichoke jars. Pour the mixture into the jars until it is about one inch from the top. Screw the lids on the jars, and with a hammer and nail, make four to eight holes in the lid. Place the jars in areas where you have ants, and watch them line up in rows to march in. Keep away from children.

FLIES Keep the kitchen clean with food put away. Screens are essential to keeping flies out. Fly swatters and flypaper—those sticky spiral bands of paper that hang from ceilings—are adequate for minor fly invasions. Make sure flypaper is not impregnated with toxic pesticide and keep it away from children.

If you have a serious fly infestation, make a citrus peel spray by simmering six to eight citrus rinds in one to two quarts of water for two to three hours, refilling as it evaporates. Cool, strain into a spray bottle, and spray areas of infestation. Citrus oils may stain cloth curtains, so test first. Keep citrus peel spray away from cats.

COCKROACHES Boric acid, a material derived from borax, has a low toxicity for humans. Available in hardware stores, boric acid powder works effectively to kill cockroaches. It can be put in floor cracks and in many hard-to-reach areas. Just make sure that the white powder cannot be ingested by pets or children.

It can take five to ten days for the boric acid to kill the roaches. If you have cockroaches, make sure that you have a can or bucket with a secure top for kitchen food scraps. Seal any cracks in the walls and floors, and eliminate water sources by fixing leaky plumbing, leaving the sink empty, and pouring out pets' water bowls at night.

GRANARY WEEVILS As mentioned in Step 7, granary weevils—grain moths—are repelled by bay leaves. Tape the leaves onto the top of cereal and rice boxes, or place them inside canisters of flour and other grains.

PROFESSIONAL PEST CONTROL If you have an infestation that you believe requires professional pest control, choose the company with care. Green Pro and Green

Healthy for You

MAKE A NATURAL FLY STRIP

1. Combine equal parts honey, sugar, and water in a saucepan.
2. Boil the mixture, stirring occasionally, until thick.
3. Remove from heat and let cool.
4. Cut strips of brown packing tape, punch a hole on one end, and loop a piece of string through the hole.
5. Dip the strips in the thick honey mixture and hang outside to dry, about 30 minutes.
6. Hang the strips in the area of worst infestation, and replace as often as needed.

Shield are certification programs for pest control service providers. Customers should be sure to ask for certified services. You may also want to contact the Rachel Carson Council for their free questionnaire for interviewing pest control specialists.

Least toxic alternatives used by a professional could include special applications of diatomaceous earth, silica aerogel, or boric acid; the use of nematodes that eat termites; or the application of heat or electric currents.

Dealing with Garbage

Our human footprint doesn't disappear after we buy and consume things; the final impact occurs when we discard items. And Americans discard a lot: about 1,600 pounds of trash per person per year. In 2006, the trash disposal rate was 4.6 pounds per person per day. Sixty-five percent came from residences; 35 percent came from schools and commercial locations such as hospitals and businesses.

Where does it all end up? About 55 percent gets buried in landfills, 33 percent gets recycled, and 12.5 percent goes to incinerators. Collecting and transporting trash and recyclables is a mammoth task. According to the National Solid Waste Management Association, the solid-waste industry employs 368,000 people. They use 148,000 vehicles to move garbage to 1,754 landfills and 87 incinerators. They also pick up recyclables at curbside in 8,660 communities and take them to 545 materials recovery facilities for sorting. Solid waste is big business, with about $47 billion in annual revenue.

It's obvious from these numbers that something has got to change—and it's got to start at home. We've got to rethink what we bring into our homes, taking into account not just how we use it but what happens to it afterward.

What you can recycle, of course, is determined at the local level. Check online or call your local recycling center. Most have brochures and clear guidelines to follow. Many also schedule special days to recycle equipment such as old toaster ovens, televisions, and computer monitors.

FOOD WASTE If you collect food scraps for composting, you know how much food waste a family can actually create in a day. Those carrot tops and onion peels add up! Some estimate that a full 10 percent of our overall garbage is food scraps—more in vegetarian families. One thing you can do to reduce your food waste is to make vegetable stock with leftover vegetable scraps. The broth will be wonderful, and nourishing in soups.

Or you can compost it.

Before the first frost, transplant your herbs into flower pots and put in a sunny kitchen window for the winter. How lovely to pick some rosemary for a mid-winter dinner, or basil for a late fall pesto.

Composting

Carrot tops, onion skins, orange peels, and even coffee grounds can be put outside in a pile or bin, then covered with grass, leaves, and brush to decompose into a rich, dirtlike organic material full of nutrients that makes excellent soil fertilizer. It is called compost—and you can keep adding layers of fruit and vegetable matter, covering it with leaves and grass, and making the compost bin or pile your main place to discard food waste.

FOUR STEPS TO COMPOSTING

- Choose a composting bin. Available in hardware stores and mail-order catalogs everywhere, composters come in a variety of designs, from a simple wooden slatted box to a large tumbler barrel. Gardening magazines are full of advertisements for composters. If you live in the country and have a lot of wild animals, look for

I'm at the age where food has taken the place of sex in my life. In fact, I've just had a mirror put over my kitchen table.

—RODNEY DANGERFIELD

an animal-resistant variety of composter. If you use compost for your own garden, and it is a large garden, consider a tumbler-barrel composter, which can make usable compost in two weeks.

- Choose a spot for your compost and a system for getting it to the composter. Make sure the compost bin is downwind from your house, at a distance far enough to keep odors away. Be careful not to keep food waste in your kitchen for very long, because molds grow very quickly on it, a serious issue for anyone with mold allergies. Keep a colander in your sink, or a bucket with a tightly covered top, to store food waste for no more than a day or two. Do not put animal products in the compost.
- The commonly used composting mixture is four parts green compost to two parts brown compost. Green compost consists of food scraps, weeds, grass cuttings, and green trimmings, and it is high in nitrogen. Brown compost consists of dead leaves, branches, brush, straw, and wood shavings, and it is high in carbon. Every time you place green compost in the pile, add half as much brown compost on top.
- Mix your compost regularly. If you turn the pile once or twice a week, the compost will decompose faster and not smell as much.

Use your compost to fertilize gardens, trees, and plants. If you don't use it yourself, many a gardener would be happy to have it. Some farmers may take fresh kitchen scraps. If you live in a city, ask farmers selling at your local market if they are interested in yours.

Plastics

Considering that plastics are made from nonrenewable petroleum and natural gas, it's not surprising that plastic manufacturing is a major source of industrial pollution. Producing a 16-ounce #1 PET bottle, for instance, generates more than a hundred times the toxic emissions to air and water as making the same size bottle out of glass. Major emissions from plastic production processes include sulfur oxides and nitrous oxides (both of which contribute to global warming) and the chemicals styrene, benzene, and trichloroethane.

Simple Stewardship

WORM COMPOSTING FOR CITY DWELLERS

If you live in a city, you can compost your garbage in a worm composting bin—no fuss, no mess.

Deborah Highly's husband gave her a worm bin for Christmas. While not high on many Christmas lists, a worm bin was what she wanted. She describes worm composting as a simple process with a few steps that people can follow in city or country.

1. Get a bin with air holes on the side, available from catalogs such as Seventh Generation and Real Goods Trading Company. (Get the worms separately; see below.) Cover the bottom of the bin with newspaper and water, in a ratio of three times more newspaper than water. (One gallon of water equals eight pounds.) If there is too little water, the worms will die.

2. You can get your worms from local gardening shops or fishing supply stores. Buy red worms. Worms from bait stores will be bigger and more expensive; little worms are more adaptive. You can also order worms by mail: They can survive for two weeks without food. Two pounds of worms will handle the food waste of a family of four to six, while one pound of worms will handle the waste from a family of two.

3. Measure your garbage. Two pounds of worms will eat one pound of garbage a day. If you overfeed the worms, the bin will begin to smell.

4. Harvest the compost in the bin every two to three months. To harvest, empty the contents of the bins by making small piles of the dirt (which is their excrement—vermicompost—and can be used as fertilizer) on newspaper and gently shaking to separate the worms.

Plastics Are Forever

When the plastics we throw away escape from garbage trucks or landfills, they get blown into trees and waterways, where they're eaten by animals that mistake them for food. In the North Pacific, a floating island of plastic waste the size of Texas has accumulated, doubling in size over the past six years. Some estimates place the load of plastic floating in that area at 3 million tons.

Nothing in nature, not even sunlight and oxygen, can break apart the bonds that hold plastic together, so it lingers on our planet indefinitely. Rather than biodegrading, plastic photodegrades into dust, winding up in soil and in the air. In bodies of water, the plastic particles absorb other harmful chemicals such as polychlorinated biphenyls (PCBs) and the pesticide DDT. Those particles then get eaten by fish, which wind up back on our dinner plates.

Despite the problems with plastic, virtually all types can be recycled a few times before becoming too weak.

TRUE TIP

A "microwave-safe" or "microwavable" label on a plastic container only means that the oven won't damage it. There is no guarantee against chemicals leaching into foods when heated. Use glass or ceramic containers instead.

Healthy for You

MAKE PACKAGING A PRIORITY

An important way to improve the environmental health of your kitchen is to carefully choose the food packaging to use.

According to a new study in the journal *Science of the Total Environment*, at least 50 chemicals found in food packaging are hormone disruptors that interfere with our bodies' natural hormone systems. The best known chemicals are bisphenol A (BPA), used in the lining of cans, and phthalates, added to plastic to make it more flexible, such as in baby bottle nipples. The study is the first to survey trace chemical residues' migration out of packaging into foods and drinks. Shoppers should take care to choose canned foods in BPA-free cans and baby bottle nipples made without phthalates.

However, confusing municipal recycling laws and limited access to recyclers who accept all types of plastic have kept recycling rates low; in 2006, a mere 6.9 percent of plastic garbage in the United States was recycled.

Hand-wash reusable containers gently with a nonabrasive soap; dishwashers and harsh detergents can scratch plastic, making hospitable homes for bacteria.

Personal Health Issues

From production through use and disposal, plastics can expose us to chemicals that are hazardous to our health, including dioxins, phthalates, and bisphenol A.

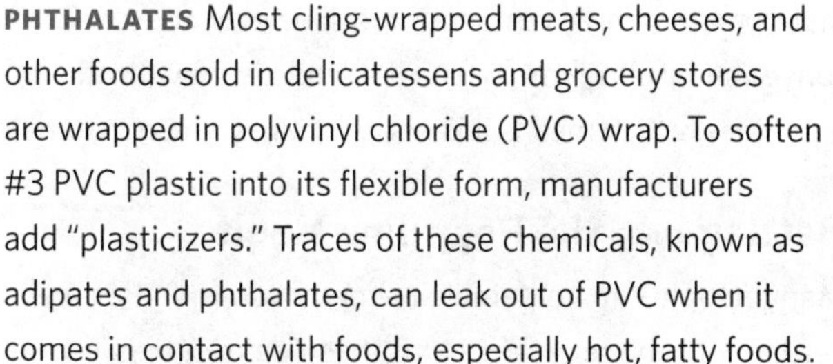

PHTHALATES Most cling-wrapped meats, cheeses, and other foods sold in delicatessens and grocery stores are wrapped in polyvinyl chloride (PVC) wrap. To soften #3 PVC plastic into its flexible form, manufacturers add "plasticizers." Traces of these chemicals, known as adipates and phthalates, can leak out of PVC when it comes in contact with foods, especially hot, fatty foods.

But adipates and phthalates have been shown to cause birth defects and damage to the liver, kidneys, lungs, and reproductive systems in mice. Phthalates are also suspected of interfering with hormones and the reproductive development of baby boys.

BISPHENOL A Many plastic items—#7 polycarbonate bottles (including baby bottles), microwave ovenware, eating utensils, as well as the plastic lining inside metal cans—are made with bisphenol A (BPA). Many studies have found that BPA interferes with hormones, as phthalates do; and a 1998 study in the journal *Environmental Health Perspectives* reported that BPA simulates the action of estrogen in human breast cancer cells. A growing number of scientists are concluding, based on animal tests, that exposure to BPA raises risks of heart disease, obesity, diabetes, and childhood behavioral problems such as hyperactivity.

Avoid storing fatty foods, such as meat and cheese, in plastic containers or plastic wrap. When purchasing cling-wrapped food from the supermarket or deli, slice off a thin layer where the food came into contact with the plastic and store the rest in a glass or ceramic container or wrap it in non-PVC cling wrap.

PLANT-BASED PLASTICS New containers and packaging made from a corn-based polymer known as polylactide (PLA) can be composted—though at very high temperatures, not in your kitchen bin. Still, it's a hopeful alternative to the 100 billion plastic bags tossed out each year and the 1.5 million tons of petroleum-based plastic used in bottles annually worldwide. PLA requires 25 to 55 percent less fossil fuels to produce than does plastic derived from petroleum, and it decomposes in 47 to 90 days, so long as it's composted in commercial facilities that operate at high temperatures. However, the conventional corn from which it's made is grown with pesticides, which means it is not an entirely green material.

Getting Into the Recycling Habit

Many people—many families—many communities are getting into the recycling habit these days. It began with newspaper and glass, then expanded to metals, and now it even extends to plastics in many localities.

And as more people turn their trash into recyclables, the market force for finding more ways to use it economically will increase.

Recycling metal is one of the most satisfying of the recycling activities, because so much of the original metal can be reclaimed. The business of metal recycling is also one to support; one California company recycles over 100 million pounds of metal a year, and provides solid jobs while doing so.

Further, if you recycle your aluminum cans you can make some money, too.

ALUMINUM Aluminum beer and soft drink containers were recovered at a rate of about 45 percent of generation (about 0.7 million tons) in 2007, and 36 percent of all aluminum in containers and packaging was recovered for recycling in 2007.

Healthy for You

DEFENSIVE SHOPPING

Bisphenol A (BPA) is an industrial compound that is commonly used to strengthen plastic and line food cans. More than one hundred peer-reviewed studies have found it to be toxic at low doses. Studies by the Center for Disease Control found BPA in the urine of 95 percent of adults sampled in 1988-94 and in 93 percent of children and adults tested in 2003-04. Canned foods are thought to be the predominant route of BPA exposure. The Environmental Working Group (EWG) tested foods and beverages from nearly one hundred cans purchased in grocery stores in three states. EWG tested 1 to 6 samples each of 28 different types of foods, including canned fruits, vegetables, pasta, beans, infant formula, meal replacements, and canned milk. BPA levels varied from less than the detection limit to a maximum level of 385 micrograms BPA per kilogram of food (one part per billion). What can you do?

- Buy prepared foods in jars when possible—especially tomatoes and tomato sauce.
- Opt for fresh produce when you can; choose frozen produce over canned.
- Use dried beans instead of canned beans.

An aluminum can that is recovered for recycling reappears back in the consumer stream in a short period of time. It takes about six weeks total to manufacture, fill, sell, recycle, and then remanufacture a beverage can. Most of the aluminum recovered from the waste stream is used to manufacture new cans, closing the loop for can production. The average aluminum can contains 40 percent post-consumer recycled aluminum.

Remove bottle caps and plastic bottle collars before recycling milk jugs and water bottles. They are made of plastic #5, not currently recycled.

Recovering aluminum for recycling saves money and dramatically reduces energy consumption. The aluminum can recycling process saves 95 percent of the energy needed to produce aluminum from bauxite ore, as well

Plastics

NUMBER	NAME	ABBREVIATION	FOUND IN
1	**Polyethylene terephthalate**	PET or PETE	Disposable soft drink, juice, and water bottles; boil-in-a-bag foods; liquid cleaning product containers; cosmetics containers.
2	**High density polyethylene**	HDPE	Gallon jugs; bottles for housecleaning items, automotive products, and cosmetics; tubs for butter and other dairy products; grocery bags.
3	**Polyvinyl chloride**	PVC	Meat wrap; bottles for cosmetics, shampoo, mouthwash, etc.; bottles for salad dressing, mineral water, cooking oil, etc.; floor-wax bottles; plumbing pipes.
4	**Low density polyethylene**	LDPE	Cling wrap, grocery bags, sandwich bags, plastic squeeze bottles, cosmetics bottles.
5	**Polypropylene**	PP	Cloudy plastic water bottles; yogurt cups and tubs; foods packaged hot, such as syrups; caps on plastic jars and bottles.
6	**Polystyrene**	PS	Disposable hot beverage cups and plates; clamshell take-out containers; egg cartons; packing peanuts.
7	**Polycarbonate**	PC	Baby bottles, some reusable water bottles, stain-resistant food storage containers, aseptic packaging.
7	**Polylactide**	PLA	Grocery bags, food containers, disposable dishware and utensils.
7	**BPA-free Plastics**		Specially labeled baby bottles and reusable water bottles.

RECYCLABLE?	RECYCLED USES	USE OR AVOID?
Yes	Textiles, fiber, twine, insulation. Also recycled into plastic containers, bottles, paintbrushes, and scouring pads.	Fine for single use. Widely accepted for recycling. Do not reuse bottles, which are hard to clean and can harbor bacteria.
Yes	Trash bins, traffic cones, plastic lumber, base cups for soft drink containers, crates, flowerpots, and more.	Use if you must. Not known to transmit chemicals into food; generally recyclable.
Yes, but do not combine with other plastics.	Construction pipes, such as for drainage and sewer; vinyl floor tiles; house siding; truck-bed liners.	Avoid if you can. Contains phthalates, which interfere with hormonal development; manufacture and incineration release dioxin, a potent carcinogen and hormone disruptor.
Yes, but not always accepted by recycling centers.		Use if you must. Not known to transmit chemicals into food; less often accepted by recycling centers.
Yes, but not always accepted by recycling centers.		Use if you must. Not known to transmit chemicals into food; less often accepted by recycling centers.
Some businesses reuse packing peanuts.	Plastic lumber	Avoid if you can. Polystyrene-foam cups and clear plastic take-out containers can leach styrene, a possible human carcinogen, into food.
Yes	Plastic lumber, paper	Avoid if you can. Made with bisphenol A, which may be linked to health problems including heart disease and obesity.
Not recyclable but compostable at high temperatures.		Use if you must. Some PLAs made from renewable resources: corn, sugarcane, potatoes.
		Choose plastic containers labeled BPA-free to avoid the risks involved with bisphenol A.

as natural resources, according to studies conducted by the Aluminum Association. The aluminum can recycling process saves 95 percent of the energy needed to produce aluminum from virgin bauxite ore, as well as natural resources, according to the Aluminum Association.

Because aluminum can be recycled, the amount of raw material needed to make the same product has shrunk in recent years. In addition, data from the Aluminum Association shows that the weight of aluminum cans has decreased by 52 percent since 1972—29 cans can be made from a pound of aluminum, up from 22 cans in 1972—and the industry continues lightening the weight of its products.

STEEL More often these days, steel recyclables are collected at curbside, drop-off sites, or multimaterial buyback centers. But there are other steel items that present bigger recycling problems, literally. Major home appliances, often referred to collectively as "white

Cooking & Eating

MAKE YOUR OWN FRIDGE SALAD BAR

Imagine your fridge with 8-10 pint and quart mason jars packed full of cut vegetables for snacks and salads. When you come home from shopping at the market and farmers' markets, or come inside with bounty from the garden, take the time to wash and cut all the vegetables and store them in the fridge all ready to eat. This system is the best chance you'll get to inspire family members to eat nine fruits and vegetables a day. The vegetable snacks are as easy to grab as chips. Try celery, carrots, red/yellow/orange peppers, artichoke hearts in a marinade, black olives, cucumbers, tomatoes, green beans, and more.

goods," have long useful lives, typically 10 to 18 years. But when they finally wear out and must be replaced, old appliances take on new value as an important source of manufacturing raw materials—scrap steel, for instance. Did you know that discarded appliances are second only to old automobiles as sources for recycled metal materials, particularly steel?

Recycling steel has a positive impact on the environment, since it takes four times as much energy to manufacture steel from virgin ore as it does to make the same steel from recycled scrap. In turn, this economy also reduces the volume of greenhouse gases released into the air during the processing and manufacturing of steel from virgin ore. Because it represents a cost savings to use recovered steel to manufacture new steel products, industrialists have an incentive to promote steel recovery, thus ensuring higher recycling rates.

Check with your local waste management office to find out whether you should leave your old appliances curbside or bring them to drop-off sites or multimaterial buyback centers. If it's a refrigerator you are recycling, be sure to ask whether the recycling center has the equipment to recycle both Freon and chlorofluorocarbons (CFCs) properly. Nearly 85 percent of CFCs in refrigerators are contained in their insulating foam, and a recycling company needs the appropriate equipment to process it safely.

The perfect kitchen gadget for making homemade tomato sauce, applesauce, and preserves is the Squeezo Strainer. Made the same as it was some 30 years ago and still made in the USA, the Best Products Squeezo Strainer is the same as the old Garden Way Squeezo Strainer later made by Lemra Products.

PAPER Processing paper from virgin timber is tough on the environment. Clear cutting can destroy wildlife habitat and increase erosion and sedimentation of streams. The cut wood is then ground, pressed, dried, and chlorine-bleached, producing more than a thousand different organochlorines, including the carcinogen dioxin and mercury. The process also requires large amounts of energy and contributes as much as 9 percent of total manufacturing carbon emissions in the United

States. At the other end of its life cycle, much of the paper we buy ends up in landfills.

The good news is that paper recycling in the United States is on the rise. Paper now accounts for more than a third of all recyclables by weight collected in the U.S. Nearly 44 million tons of paper and paperboard were recovered in 2006—a recycling rate of over 50 percent. By 2012, the paper industry hopes to recover 60 percent of the paper Americans consume. Every ton of paper recycled saves more than 3.3 cubic yards of landfill space.

GLASS According to the EPA, Americans sent 13.6 million tons of glass into the municipal solid waste stream in 2007. About 24 percent of that glass was recovered for recycling. That number seems low, but it's a significant improvement: Glass recovery in the U.S. increased from 750,000 tons in 1980 to more than 3.2 million tons in 2007.

Soft drink, beer, food, wine, and liquor containers represent the largest source of glass generated and

Simple Stewardship

GREENING YOUR KITCHEN

Consider this your checklist:

- Choose safer products for cleaning
- Choose integrated pest man agement and non-toxic controls
- Integrate water-conservation practices
- Recycle and compost
- Practice energy efficiency
- Choose healthy cookware and food packaging
- Establish healthy cabinets and structures
- Establish a place for house hold hazardous waste removal

SNAPSHOT **WILL ALLEN**

"We want to teach young people how to grow the soil, how to grow the food, how to harvest, wash and package food, and how to eat it."

Milwaukee, WI

Founder and CEO, Growing Power National Training and Community Food Center in Milwaukee

Feeding an estimated 10,000 people with produce grown on urban farms in Wisconsin and Illinois, Growing Power combines aquaculture and agriculture to provide fish and fresh vegetables to local communities living in urban food deserts. The program works in a closed loop by collecting waste from tilapia (or lake perch) to serve as fertilizer for the produce.

At the heart of Growing Power is its youth corps program. Allen himself was the son of a sharecropper who left the South but wanted to be sure his sons knew how to farm. After a pro basketball career and sales work, Allen returned to farming with the purchase of a two-acre lot in Milwaukee.

recovered for recycling. Glass in durable goods, such as furniture, appliances, and especially consumer electronics, rounds out the sources of postconsumer glass.

The glass containing your soda today might be the glass containing your spaghetti sauce tomorrow. That's because glass, especially glass food and beverage containers, can be recycled over and over again. In fact, 90 percent of recycled glass is used to make new containers. Other uses for recycled glass include kitchen tiles, counter tops, and wall insulation. Glass makers have always known the material's recyclability, but glass recycling has grown considerably in recent years. This growth is due to both increased collection through curbside recycling programs and glass manufacturers' increased demand for recycled glass.

To recycle glass, wash it thoroughly, inside and out. Remove paper labels if possible. Remove any jar or bottle tops.

A Few Final Words

True Food began years ago. It grew out of *The Green Kitchen Handbook,* written by Annie B. Bond and the staff of Mothers & Others for a Livable Planet, a nonprofit established by Wendy Gordon and Meryl Streep.

That book, and now this one, owe much to a 1986 article in the *Journal of Nutrition Education* titled "Dietary Guidelines for Sustainability," written by Joan Dye Gussow, professor of nutrition and education at Teachers College, Columbia University, and Kate Clancy, professor of nutrition and food service management at Syracuse University.

In their article, Gussow and Clancy introduced the term "sustainable diets," and they recommended food choices that, in addition to answering human nutritional needs, support the life and health of Earth's natural systems into the foreseeable future.

Stir-Fried Collard Greens

Thanks to Will Allen's Growing Power National Training and Community Food Center, urban youth in Wisconsin and Illinois are growing as well as eating their vegetables. His work, and his recipes, give new meaning to the term soul food. SERVES 2 TO 4 PEOPLE

1 to 2 pounds collard greens
3 tablespoons olive oil (or equal amounts butter and olive oil)
Salt and pepper

1. Thoroughly wash collard greens.
2. Roll up greens and dice them.
3. Heat olive oil in a frying pan over medium heat. Add diced greens.
4. Salt and pepper to taste. (You can also add a little honey.)
5. Stir fry for about 15 minutes, less if you prefer greens with more of a raw crunch.

Now, years later, the subject of food and our out-of-true food system is front page news. No one then would have imagined the First Lady planting an organic kitchen garden on the White House lawn, nor crowds going to mainstream movie theaters to view films like *Fast Food Nation, Food, Inc.*, and *Supersize Me.* It's a whole new world we live in, when giants like Wal-Mart boast that they are the largest purveyors of organic food and advocate local sourcing, and when the Secretary of Agriculture contemplates ways to expand the farm-to-school program to provide fresh, whole, and healthy foods from regional farmers to school children in urban areas.

The three of us have joyfully collaborated to make *True Food* a guidebook on how to put big ideas into everyday practice in a way that brings pleasure, not pain, and joy and connection, not suffering.

True food nourishes us physically and emotionally, in ways profound, beyond basic sustenance. When we eat food that is true to its nature, we give our bodies the pure nutrients required for maximum health—and we allow ourselves a connection to the environment in a way that industrialized food does not allow. We become part of a natural ecosystem, one that is sustainable and that promises no end to the pleasures of eating.

The kitchen is a country in which there are always discoveries to be made.

—**GRIMOD DE LA REYNIERE (CIRCA 1800)**

Index

P

About the Authors

ANNIE B. BOND is a best-selling author who has been helping people live greener and healthier lives for over 20 years. She is the author of five books in the field, including *Better Basics for the Home, Clean & Green,* and *Home Enlightenment*. She is the editor of numerous green magazines and websites and has written thousands of articles in the areas of natural lifestyles and green household care. Currently she is editor-in-chief and CEO of Green Chi Cafe, a media site for sharing the culture of green. She lives in Rhinebeck, New York.

MELISSA BREYER is a writer and editor specializing in sustainable food, cooking, and health. She has edited and written for regional, national, and international books and periodicals, and her work has appeared in the *New York Times Magazine* and the *Green Market Baking Book*. Breyer is senior editor of Healthy and Green Living for Care2, a worldwide natural lifestyles social network and website with ten million members. She writes about food and creates new recipes daily for the site. She lives in Brooklyn, New York.

WENDY GORDON cofounded Mothers & Others for a Livable Planet, a pioneering consumer outreach organization, in 1989, and went on to establish *Green Guide,* the go-to resource for the eco-conscious consumer, acquired in 2007 by National Geographic. Mothers & Others was conceived at the Natural Resources Defense Council (NRDC), where Gordon was a senior project scientist in the health program. She now serves as a consultant for the NRDC's communications department, guiding the next-phase development of its consumer action portal, Simple Steps, and its new web resource for communities, Smarter Cities. She lives in New York City.

ALICE WATERS, chef and proprietor of Chez Panisse in Berkeley, California, is an American culinary pioneer and a passionate advocate for a food economy that is good, clean, and fair. She established the Chez Panisse Foundation in 1996 to support the Edible Schoolyard, a model public education program whose success led to the School Lunch Initiative, integrating a nutritious daily lunch and gardening experience into the academic curriculum of all public schools in the United States. Waters is vice president of Slow Food International and the author of eight books, including *The Art of Simple Food: Notes and Recipes from a Delicious Revolution.*

TRUE FOOD

by Annie B. Bond, Melissa Breyer, and Wendy Gordon

How to Save Seeds, page 67, used by permission of Seed Savers Exchange.

Snapshot: Dan Barber, pages 74-75, excerpted from "You Say Tomato, I Say Agricultural Disaster" by Dan Barber, *New York Times,* August 8, 2009. Used by permission of the *New York Times.*

Genetic Diversity & Our Future, page 80, used by permission of Cary Fowler.

ISBN 978-1-4262-0727-3 (special sale edition)

Library of Congress Cataloging-in-Publication Data

Berthold-Bond, Annie.
True food : 8 simple steps to a healthier you / Annie B. Bond, Melissa Breyer, Wendy Gordon.
p. cm.
Includes index.
ISBN 978-1-4262-0594-1
1. Nutrition. 2. Sustainable living. I. Breyer, Melissa, 1957- II. Gordon, Wendy, 1957- III. Title.
RA784.B396 2010
613.2--dc22

2009041965

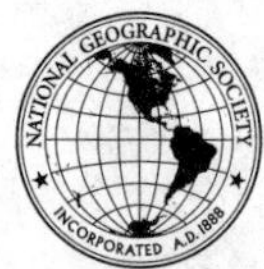

The National Geographic Society is one of the world's largest nonprofit scientific and educational organizations. Founded in 1888 to "increase and diffuse geographic knowledge," the Society works to inspire people to care about the planet. It reaches more than 325 million people worldwide each month through its official journal, *National Geographic,* and other magazines; National Geographic Channel; television documentaries; music; radio; films; books; DVDs; maps; exhibitions; school publishing programs; interactive media; and merchandise. National Geographic has funded more than 9,000 scientific research, conservation and exploration projects and supports an education program combating geographic illiteracy.

For more information, please call 1-800-NGS LINE (647-5463) or write to the following address:

National Geographic Society
1145 17th Street N.W.
Washington, D.C. 20036-4688 U.S.A.

Visit us online at www.nationalgeographic.com

For information about special discounts for bulk purchases, please contact National Geographic Books Special Sales: ngspecsales@ngs.org

For rights or permissions inquiries, please contact National Geographic Books Subsidiary Rights: ngbookrights@ngs.org

BOOK DESIGN: Chalkley Calderwood

Printed in U.S.A.

15/CW-CML/1